W9-CSI-078

CONTENTS

INTRODUCTION

This is a book written for parents about many common childhood illnesses. It is not meant to be an encyclopedia of pediatrics that describes all the diseases of childhood. Nor is it intended to be a manual of first aid.

I am trying to talk to concerned mothers and fathers in a calm and easy-to-understand style. After many years of practicing pediatrics and public health, I believe that most parents want to know the basic and practical information about various ailments of infants and children. They are interested in short descriptions of many childhood diseases, their causes, and their key symptoms. They need to become aware of serious symptoms and to learn when to call the doctor for advice or examination. It is also helpful for parents to understand some medical terms used in pediatric illnesses so that they can speak a "common language" with their child's doctor.

When a child is sick, the physician's responsibility is to make a proper diagnosis and to prescribe appropriate treatment. However, in order to do his job, he must rely on the child's parents to do their job. Parents play a vital role in detecting early signs of illness, providing a clear description of symptoms, and following through with treatment. Parents are also responsible for the daily routines that help to maintain a child's health and in many cases, they can take preventive measures against various illnesses. What I'm describing here is essentially teamwork between the child's doctor and the child's parents.

In this book, I emphasize information I believe parents need to know in order to do their job and focus on the prevention of diseases and the alleviation of symptoms. For communicable diseases such as chicken pox and strep throat, I discuss such things as how long the disease is contagious and when a sick child can safely return to his school or daycare activities. But I avoid discussion of the diagnosis and treatment of diseases.

In preparing this book, I carefully researched several current, authoritative textbooks of pediatrics, in addition to the most recent publications of the American Academy of Pediatrics and the American Public Health Association for factual material. My goal was to provide a quick and easy reference guide for parents of infants and children. I have provided thumbnail summaries of the most common illnesses and offer only a minimum of technical details of each illness. Each key ends with two sections: "What Parents Can Do" and "What the Doctor May Do." The first gives parents direct advice about dealing with the illness, and the second helps parents know what to expect from their child's doctor.

I would like readers to know that my coauthor is my daughter. As a clinical psychologist and a new mother, she added a fresh perspective to the text. She reminded me how upsetting it can be for parents when their child is ill and how a little information at the right time can go a long way.

If I can reduce some parental anxieties and misconceptions about the cause and course of many childhood illnesses, one of my goals will be reached. If I can reassure you as a parent that your child can cope well with many illnesses—in some cases with the aid of the physician and in some cases without such aid—another goal will be reached. As you and your child grow older, experience will become your best instructor.

Norman B. Schell, M.D.   May 26, 1992

1

TUNING IN TO SIGNS OF ILLNESS

Early in their medical training, physicians learn that taking a good history from a sick patient can help make the right diagnosis at least 75 percent of the time. That's why your doctor will ask you several key questions when you bring your sick child to him. His questions will include: "When did you first notice your child (vomiting, having diarrhea, coughing, running a fever)? How many times a day did these things occur?" Your answers to these questions will give the doctor a handle on the onset, duration, and frequency of your child's symptoms. These facts are called a *history* and can prove very helpful in the diagnosis.

Let's begin with a common example. In order for you to give an accurate history, you must carefully observe your child every day during her illness. Watch for symptoms such as loss of appetite, irritability, fatigue, flushed face, coughing, or runny nose. The loss of appetite is often the very first sign of sickness. If your child has symptoms such as sore throat, headache, earache, diarrhea, or muscle pains, you should make a mental or written note about what is happening and when. You can then give an accurate history when the doctor examines her.

The next step is to check your child's body temperature with an oral or rectal thermometer, depending on her age. If your child is over six years old, use the oral (under-the-tongue) thermometer; otherwise, use the rectal one. (Be sure you learn how to use a thermometer and how to read it before she becomes ill.)

If a rectal thermometer reads over 100°F (Fahrenheit), your child has a fever. If you are using an oral thermometer, any temperature reading over 99°F can be called a fever. If she does not have a fever, don't take her temperature more than every three or four hours unless her body becomes very warm to the touch. Keep a written record of the date, time, and reading whenever you take it. These records may prove extremely useful to the doctor when you call later.

Fever occurs frequently in infants and young children. However, it does not necessarily mean that there is a serious infection. Sometimes serious infections can occur with low fever, and sometimes mild infections can occur with high fever. The height of the fever does not necessarily indicate how severe the infection is. However, a high fever needs to be managed quickly.

If your child's temperature is 104°F or above, it is considered a high fever. Try to stay calm, and call the doctor, who may advise acetaminophen (such as Tylenol®) and sponge baths in warm water. Body temperature is normally at is lowest level in the morning and rises after 4 or 5 P.M. If the thermometer reading is 102° or 103° in the morning or early afternoon, you can bet it will reach 103° or 104° in the evening. That is why it's important to call your pediatrician during the early part of the day so that an office visit can be arranged.

Some doctors don't advise the use of antifever medications such as acetaminophen unless the fever is high. Their idea is that a fever is one of the body's natural defense mechanisms to fight bacterial and viral infections. Other doctors hold off on antifever medications because they don't want to suppress a low-grade fever to normal and "hide" the appearance of a true infection in the body. They prefer to observe the natural course of the disease with thermometer readings taken every three or four hours. Ask your doctor what her policy is.

Carefully observe your child for any change in her symptoms or behavior. Is the diarrhea or the vomiting becoming more frequent? Is she becoming more irritable, restless, or drowsy? Is her headache or bellyache worsening? Does she have fever? Is it rising? If any of these things are happening, don't hesitate to keep the doctor informed or to bring your child to the office for an examination.

Remember: you have an essential role in detecting early signs of illness in your child. The pediatrician is the expert, but nobody knows your child as well as you do. Your doctor will rely on you to report changes in your child's behavior, to describe symptoms, and to follow through with treatment at home. Parents also play a critical role in comforting and easing the pain of their sick child. The more familiar you become with various childhood illnesses, the more at ease you will be in dealing with them. One of the first things you need to know is which conditions signal a medical emergency for your child.

Call the doctor quickly if any of the following occur:

- Temperature over 104°F
- Difficulty breathing (go to the nearest emergency room)
- Bluish discoloration of lips (go to the nearest emergency room)
- Pulling inward of chest wall with each breath (retractions)
- Wheezing or noisy breath sounds
- Loud, croupy cough with a hoarse cry

3

- Marked drowsiness or listlessness
- Muscular twitching or jerking (convulsions)
- Severe pain in abdomen, head, or ear
- Watery bowel movements every one or two hours
- Repeated, projectile ("shooting out") vomiting
- Continuous crying (infants)

Regardless of whether your child has fever, call the doctor whenever she looks and acts sick.

2

~~~~~~

BACTERIAL AND VIRAL INFECTIONS

We're all surrounded by a wide variety of bacteria and viruses in our daily environment. You might say the entire world is covered with a thin layer of microscopic organisms of one kind or another. Fortunately, most of them do not cause diseases. Healthy infants and children, like healthy adults, don't usually become ill whenever they come in contact with many common bacteria and virus. Illnesses usually require a hefty dose of powerful bacteria or viruses.

What are Bacteria and Viruses?

Bacteria are microscopic, single-celled living organisms. To see bacteria clearly, microscopes with magnifications of 1,000 times or more are needed. Bacteria have different shapes and forms and are found in soil, air, natural waters, vegetation, dust, and food products. Large numbers of "friendly" (i.e., harmless) bacteria normally live on our skin, in our nose and throat, and in our intestinal tract. However, it is not natural to have bacteria of any kind living in any other healthy tissue or organ of the body.

Some bacteria normally live in large numbers on everybody's skin surface, but they don't cause infection unless they enter cut or broken skin. Most disease-causing organisms are parasites of humans or animals that invade the body and grow within the tissues. Some types do damage by penetrating cells, but most do damage by multiplying outside the cells.

Viruses are much smaller than bacteria and can only be seen under electron microscopes. They can survive only a short time outside the human cells. This makes it more difficult to "catch" some viral infections than bacterial infections.

Infection

An infection occurs in your child when bacteria or viruses enter her body and settle in a local area like the skin, nose, throat, or intestines. Interestingly, the body's environment (temperature, food supply, etc.) helps to promote the rapid growth of these tiny organisms. Some types of bacteria, such as staph and strep, can double in number every half hour for the first several hours after they take hold. However, it usually takes some time before you can notice the signs and symptoms of an infectious disease.

The *incubation period* is the time interval between the first contact with disease-causing bacteria (or a virus) and the appearance of the first signs or symptoms of the disease. If you want to trace where (or from whom) your child caught a disease, ask your doctor about the incubation period for that particular disease.

It's also important to know how long your child is contagious. Sometimes, even though signs of a disease are still present, there is no longer a danger of passing it along to another child. For example, my granddaughter recently had a case of roseola, a common illness among babies that usually includes a high fever and a pinkish rash. Once the rash appeared, her disease was no longer contagious, and she was able to go out and socialize as usual.

Bodily Resistance

Even after being exposed to disease-causing organisms, your child may not become ill. This happens because the body contains many built-in tools and techniques that fight off the invasion or growth of bacteria and viruses. This resistance, or immunity to infections, can be either short-lived or long-lasting. An important means of acquiring immunity is through immunization, that is, "shots" your doctor administers on regular, wellness visits. Specific immunizations at prescribed intervals are needed in order for your child to develop long-lasting *antibodies*, which are protective protein substances circulating in the body. Another way of acquiring immunity is through past infections (illnesses) with specific bacteria (or viruses). Chickenpox is an example of an illness that children usually have only once because of long-lasting immunity.

There are many defensive mechanisms in the blood and tissues that can prevent or fight off infections. Infants and children have many of these general resistance mechanisms in their blood and tissues. For the first few months of their life, they also have many specific antibodies transferred to them from their mother during pregnancy. After that time, they need to receive specific immunizations in order to develop their own long-lasting antibodies.

Your child will contact many bacteria in soil and dirt and in uncooked food, but most of these organisms are harmless to her skin or to her intestines if swallowed (in small amounts); because her skin and mouth and stomach contain antibacterial substances (such as acids and enzymes) that usually can ward off or kill the bacteria. However, if dirt enters a cut or scrape on her skin, the skin must be thoroughly cleaned and an antiseptic solution applied.

Antibiotics
Particular antibiotics work best against particular bacteria infections. Very few antibiotics work against viral infections. Antibiotics have different ways of attacking bacteria;

some stop the continuous growth of bacteria but allow some to survive for a while until the body's own defense system can destroy them, whereas others kill bacteria directly.

Some antibiotics are most effective against a limited number of disease-causing bacteria. Those antibiotics that work on a wide range of disease-causing bacteria are known as broad-spectrum antibiotics. If a specimen from an infected site such as the throat or an abscess is taken and sent to a microbiology laboratory, the specific bacteria can be identified and the laboratory can test a variety of antibiotics against them to find out which is most likely to cure the infection. This procedure is called *culture and sensitivity testing*.

Often an antibiotic that was found effective in sensitivity testing may become ineffective in the course of prolonged treatment. Such drug resistance usually occurs when the bacteria develop new strains (variants) that are able to cope with the antibiotic. In these cases, the antibiotic has to be changed to a more effective one as shown by further sensitivity tests on the laboratory cultures.

What Parents Can Do

- Call the doctor when your child has a high fever (103°F or above) or has a low fever for more than a day. Report not only the temperature but the method taken (oral or rectal).
- If you are using antibiotics, administer them to your child for the full amount of time prescribed.
- Keep an up-to-date record of your child's immunizations and illnesses.
- Don't have your child play with another who is ill.
- Reduce your child's exposure to illness by avoiding indoor crowds when possible.
- Wash toys, especially if you have an infant. Children of this age like to put their toys and others' toys in the mouth.

- Wash your hands and your child's hands frequently. Having clean hands is one way to reduce the spread of disease-causing germs.
- Keep cuts clean, and apply an antiseptic and a sterile adhesive strip daily.

What the Doctor May Do

- Prescribe antibiotics
- Take a throat culture if your child develops a sore throat with a fever. This is done before antibiotics are given.
- Take a stool culture if your child has diarrhea with fever for several days. This is done to rule out a bacterial infection of the intestines.

3

~~~~~~

ABDOMINAL PAINS

Abdominal pain ("bellyache") is a very common complaint in children of all ages, like the common headache complaint of adults. Your infant can't point to his abdomen and tell you where it hurts. But if she cries loudly for a long period, bends her legs up, and passes gas, she probably has a bellyache.

Many conditions, both psychological and physical, can cause sudden or acute abdominal pain. Most of the time the pain passes quickly and means little. However, it may be important if it continues for more than two hours or if any of the following events occur with it:

- Fever
- Vomiting
- Drowsiness

If these symptoms are present, contact the doctor for her evaluation and advice.

Colic

During her first month, your infant may develop the problem known as *colic*. (Be consoled by the fact that about 20 percent of all infants have a fussy and cranky period each day—mostly in the late afternoon or evening.) She may seem to be in some pain or discomfort, and she may go on crying for hours without finding any relief in her pacifier or in burping, rocking, or lullabies. The more she cries, the more air she swallows and the more gas she'll pass. She may clench her hands, and her arms may bend tightly against her body. This regular, stressful event continues until she becomes exhausted (and you do, too). Occasionally, the passage of gas or stool may relieve it temporarily.

Even in this day of major medical discoveries, the exact cause of colic hasn't been clarified yet. Some experts believe it's due to oversensitivity to environmental stimuli. Some say it can be caused by sensitivity to protein in the milk formula or to a food in the mother's diet (in breast-fed colicky infants). Try to keep a calm attitude if your baby has colic, because tense parents can make things worse.

The doctor should examine your baby to make sure there are no other reasons for his crying spells. He may then suggest several treatments, such as new formula or medication. The good news is that colic rarely lasts more than three months, and both you and your infant will survive the ordeal.

Constipation

If your infant has a hard and dry bowel movement or moves his bowels less frequently than once a day, abdominal cramps may develop, and he may cry before or during the passage of the stools. Older children may have problems when they have hard stools after two or three days without having any movement. They too may complain of bellyaches. (See Key 11.)

Other Causes of Abdominal Pain

Sore throats caused by bacterial or viral infections, such as streptococcus (strep) or measles, may cause abdominal pains if lymph glands around the intestines become enlarged. Some pneumonias and anemias can cause belly pains, too.

Urinary tract infections in children over three years— especially girls—may cause pain within the abdomen.

11

Besides the bellyache, there may be frequent urination with pain and burning. This is discussed further in Key 33.

Intestinal infections (called *gastroenteritis*) often produce abdominal cramps or continuous pain. Viruses usually cause these infections, but bacteria or parasites can also be at the root. Viral gastroenteritis often occurs in more than one member of the family at the same time. Bacterial gastroenteritis usually comes from eating contaminated food that has been incompletely refrigerated or cooked. Diarrhea or vomiting occurs during most intestinal infections.

Appendicitis is rare under two years of age and is infrequent under 15 years. Although many cases don't follow the typical pattern, usually the first location of pain is in the center of the abdomen, and after a few hours the pain moves to the lower right side of the abdomen. Your child will probably have fever and vomiting along with the pain. It's very important to have the doctor examine him after the first couple of hours of constant pain because early diagnosis and treatment (appendectomy) will prevent complications from the infection.

Allergy to cow's milk can cause colicky pains in the abdomen of some infants and young children. A milk-substitute formula such as soybean (or lactose-free) milk may cause a dramatic cure of the bellyaches. Most children (up to 85 percent) outgrow their milk allergies by four years of age. (For more on allergies, refer to Key 5.)

Psychological tension caused by stressful events in school or at home (such as sibling rivalry or divorce or death in the family) may produce intermittent abdominal pains. Usually these bellyaches occur without any other signs of illness such as fever, diarrhea, or vomiting. At times a child may mimic another sibling or a parent who has abdominal pain episodes related to anxiety or tension.

If abdominal pains recur *regularly* for several months, they may be termed *chronic* rather than *acute*. Recurrent pains may indicate a problem in the gastrointestinal tract or in other organs in the abdomen. If your child has this type of pain history, check for loss of appetite, loss of weight, or signs of blood in the bowel movements (either bright red or pitch black). Make sure he has a complete diagnostic workup by the doctor.

When to Call the Doctor

- If your child comes down with a bellyache, take her temperature and call the doctor for advice.
- Call the doctor for an examination if she has any severe abdominal pain that causes much crying or extreme restlessness.
- Call the doctor for an examination if she has any bellyache that lasts for two or more hours continuously.
- Call the doctor for an examination if she has fever, vomiting, or drowsiness along with her abdominal pain.

What Parents Can Do

- Don't give any laxatives to relieve a bellyache unless the doctor approves.
- To relieve the stress of caring for a colicky baby, try to arrange breaks for yourself. Even a brief walk around the block by yourself can be helpful. Mobilize the support of relatives and friends.
- Make sure food is refrigerated well and cooked thoroughly as a preventive measure against bacterial gastroenteritis.
- If you suspect your child has a milk allergy, raise the possibility of switching to soy milk with your child's doctor.
- If your child has chronic bellyaches, have her checked out by the doctor. If his evaluation does not reveal any physical cause, consider psychological factors. Young children are

often unable to express feelings and instead express their emotional upset through bodily symptoms.

What the Doctor May Do

- Change the formula or diet.
- Take a blood count.
- Take a urine analysis.
- Order an x-ray of the abdomen.
- Do a rectal examination.
- Re-examine her abdomen after a couple of hours.
- If she is vomiting, advise giving her sips of cold cola soda every 15 to 29 minutes and *no* food intake.
- Observe the child in the hospital if the pain continues for a few hours.

4

~~~~~~

ADENOID AND TONSIL PROBLEMS

The tonsils are almond-shaped masses on either side of the throat. Further back, between the nose and the throat, lie the adenoid masses. They lie near the auditory (eustachian) tubes. The adenoids can be seen only by using a special mirror or by taking special soft-tissue x-rays of the *nasopharynx* (the area where the throat meets the back of the nose).

The tonsils and the adenoids contain important lymphoid tissues that are the factory and the home of white blood cells called lymphocytes. These cells ward off infections by producing many specific antibodies and specialized disease-fighting cells as part of the body's defensive system. All lymphoid tissues throughout the body normally grow in size until adolescence and then begin to shrink. The tonsils and adenoids should not bother your child unless they are large enough to interfere with his swallowing or breathing.

Tonsils can become temporarily inflamed due to infection. This condition is sometimes treated with antibiotics. (See Key 32 on tonsillitis and sore throats.) Chronic enlargement of the tonsils and the adenoids is more troublesome and can occur from normal growth, recurrent infections in the nose and throat, or allergies.

Signs of Enlargement
One sign of enlarged tonsils and adenoids is that the air-

way to the bronchial tubes and the lungs may become blocked and cause mouth breathing during the day and snoring during sleep. As you observe your child, you might notice "pulling in" (retractions) of the front of the chest or observe several seconds when breathing stops during sleep (*sleep apnea*). Because young infants breathe through the nose instead of the mouth, there can be serious consequences when the adenoids are swollen.

Occasionally, enlarged tonsils may reach a size where swallowing food becomes difficult. Enlarged adenoids can also lead to severe distortion of speech, continuous nasal discharge, or nocturnal cough. But don't be hasty in drawing conclusions, because the latter two symptoms may also be caused by other conditions, such as allergies or nose or throat infections, called upper respiratory infections. (For more on these topics, see Keys 10 and 18.)

Recurrent middle ear infections may result from enlarged adenoidal tissue blocking the eustachian tubes, the short connecting links from the nasopharynx (part of the throat behind the nasal passages) to the middle ear.

Indications for Surgery

Years ago the surgical removal of the tonsils and adenoids was routinely advised for the majority of children before they reached school age. Many doctors recommended this operation as part of standard medical care in the belief that tonsils and adenoids served no useful function. They believed that removing the tonsils and adenoids would prevent many colds and throat and ear infections. However, the results of large-scale studies conducted in many reputable hospital clinics did not support this idea. Instead, the studies showed that children who lost their tonsils and adenoids by surgery came down with just as many colds and throat and ear infections as those who still had their tonsils and adenoids.

Over the last 30 years, fewer and fewer children have had surgery to remove their tonsils and adenoids. By the 1970s most physicians were reluctant to advise the operation without having a good reason. Today there is a prevailing medical consensus that this surgery should be performed only when there are specific and sound reasons for doing so. Having frequent tonsillitis or sore throats does not necessarily warrant surgery.

In 1991 the American Academy of Pediatrics prepared an official statement recommending surgical removal of the tonsils or adenoids only if one or more of the following "urgent" conditions exists:

1. Air is blocked from reaching the lungs due to enlarged tonsils or adenoids. You may notice this if the child has breathing difficulty during the day or if breathing stops for more than 10 seconds during sleep. (This is called sleep apnea.)
2. The child experiences severe difficulty in swallowing because of enlarged tonsils.
3. There is extreme discomfort in breathing such as continuous mouth breathing during the day and loud snoring during sleep. This may involve the adenoids only.
4. There is marked nasally distorted speech due to very large adenoids. Only the adenoids may be removed to correct this condition.

Several other indications for surgical removal were made by the Academy at the same time, but they were not considered as "urgent" as the four above. They include:

• Pockets of pus (abscess) around and behind the tonsils
• Multiple middle-ear infections that continue to occur despite the use of other accepted methods of prevention and treatment.

What Parents Can Do

- Keep in mind that frequent colds, runny noses, and ear infections are usually *not* caused by problems with the tonsils or adenoids.
- If you hear your child snoring, observe whether she seems to be having difficulty breathing. Do you notice a pulling in of the chest or sleep apnea? Report these observations to your child's doctor.

What the Doctor May Do

- Examine your child's ear, nose, and throat regularly on wellness visits and especially when you report a potential problem in that area.
- Refer you to an ENT (ear, nose, and throat) specialist in order to evaluate the true status of the tonsils and adenoids.

5

‸‸‸

ALLERGIES TO FOODS

I t would not be unusual for your child to have some type of allergy, since between 10 and 20 percent of people develop one or more allergies during their lifetime. Some of these allergies are seasonal and are reactions to inhaled pollens or dust. Other allergies are triggered by certain foods. Food allergies may cause itchy rashes like hives or oozing and scaling rashes (eczema). Asthma is another type of allergy that can be very debilitating and will be discussed in detail in Key 7. Most allergies are manageable once you are able to narrow down which agent caused the reaction. This is where your record keeping may come in handy.

Do allergies run in families? Most allergic children have a history of allergies in one side of the family or the other. In fact, about 35 percent of allergic children have allergy histories in both sides of the family. When children have such a strong inheritance pattern, they are more vulnerable to severe allergic symptoms early in life. However, while these children inherit a general tendency toward food allergies, they are unlikely to inherit a specific allergy to a specific food. For example, a father may develop swollen lips and eyelids from eating chocolate, whereas his child may tolerate chocolate but break out with itchy, red blotches or bumps (hives) scattered over his body after eating strawberries.

Antigens and Antibodies
    Although not all food allergies are caused by antibodies, many allergic symptoms are caused by reactions of *antibody*

to *antigen*. You may already be familiar with these terms since antigens and antibodies play a vital role in immunizing your child against diseases. To understand their different role in the allergic process, let's use the image of soldiers in battle.

Antigens are like foreign soldiers invading the body, and antibodies are the troops sent out by the immune system to fight them off. Technically, antigens are specific protein substances introduced into the body by eating or breathing. They stimulate or sensitize certain cells (T cells and plasma cells) in the immune system to produce opposing proteins called antibodies. The antibodies continue to circulate in the blood, tissues, and skin. It's as if they "stand guard" for a long time once the antigens have been introduced into the body.

Allergic Process

The allergic child is more sensitive to the introduction of antigens. Each time he is exposed to a new antigen, his immune system manufactures the antibody to that antigen. As more of this antibody is made over time, the child becomes more allergic. It may take anywhere from weeks to years for the amount of antibody to reach a high level. It may seem as if the child has developed an allergy "overnight," but in reality the allergy is the end result of an internal process that may have been going on for some time. Once the antibody reaches a high level, symptoms may appear whenever the child comes in contact with the antigen.

When the antigen and the antibody join on the surface of specialized cells (mast cells) in the nose, skin, eyes, intestinal tract, and bronchial tubes of the lungs, these cells release several chemicals. These chemicals include histamines and other substances that cause the allergic symptoms. You can now see why many cold remedies are labeled as "antihistamines"— they are designed to block the effects of histamine.

Common Food Allergens

Allergens are specific antigens—the "foreign" substances introduced into the body that set the allergic process in motion. Almost any food can act as an allergen. The most frequent ones are: fish (especially shellfish), peanuts, eggs, chocolate, strawberries, milk, and wheat. Even small quantities of food allergens are usually enough to bring on an allergic reaction in a previously sensitized child, and the reaction can begin shortly after ingesting the allergen.

Diagnosis

You can never be certain that your child has a true food allergy unless she always reacts to that particular food after eating it. Skin (*intradermal*) tests to confirm food allergies are of little value. Many children show a positive reaction to a particular food that is injected into the skin but do not react to it when it is swallowed. The true test is the appearance of a reaction such as a rash or the swelling of the tongue or the eyelids within a few minutes to a few hours after the child swallows the food.

You can help with the "detective" work of allergic reactions by keeping a careful record of which suspected foods cause a reaction. Make note of *what kind of reaction* follows and *how much time* elapses before the reaction begins. In the case of infants and small children, it is recommended that you introduce one new food at a time so that you have the opportunity to observe whether that food causes a reaction.

Another strategy that physicians sometimes use is the "elimination diet." The suspected food is eliminated from your child's diet for seven to 14 days, and no new foods can be given during that whole period. If the allergic symptoms then disappear, the food is reintroduced to the diet to see if the same symptoms reappear within 24 hours. If the symptoms do not disappear in seven to 14 days, another suspected food has to be eliminated.

Pediatricians and allergists may occasionally recommend "provocative food challenge studies" or other tests to solve some difficult allergy puzzles. Minute amounts of suspected food allergens are fed to the child to see if they produce allergic symptoms. These food challenges must be done under carefully controlled and supervised conditions.

Management

Once your child is diagnosed as having a food allergy, the management is pretty straightforward. The suspected food or foods must be completely avoided in any amounts. If the causative food is not readily found, the doctor may prescribe antihistamines or other medications to control symptoms such as itching or swelling. *Subcutaneous* (which means under the skin) injections of food antigens known as "allergy shots" are *rarely* effective in management of food allergies. However, some food allergies may disappear over the years.

When to Call the Doctor

• If your child's allergic reaction to a food causes wheezing, difficulty breathing, or swelling of the eyelids, lips, or tongue.
• If the allergic reaction causes a severely itchy rash that interferes with sleeping or normal daily activities.

What Parents Can Do

• Introduce only one new food per week to your infant and only in gradually increasing quantities. Even with baby foods, avoid mixtures at first until you're sure your child doesn't have a problem with any of the ingredients.
• Introduce your child to new foods only when she is feeling well.

- When a specific food has been suspected by the doctor, make sure you carefully check the ingredients labels of all foods your allergic child eats for any mention of that food. No matter how small an amount may be present, it must be avoided.
- Keep a written record of each new food you introduce to your healthy infant with a notation of the date given. If a reaction seems to follow within 24 hours, make a note of it for the doctor when you call him.

What the Doctor May Do

- Advise an elimination diet in which suspected foods are eliminated from the diet and then reintroduced one at a time to see if symptoms reappear in 24 hours.
- Advise skin allergy testing by an allergist.
- Prescribe an antihistamine to control allergic symptoms.

6

ANEMIA

Many times it's hard to tell if your infant or child has *anemia*, which is a deficiency in the quantity or the quality of the blood. The symptoms can vary from none at all to pallor, tiredness, shortness of breath, or rapid heart beat. The symptoms depend on the severity of the anemia, the type of anemia, and how long your child has had it.

Anemia that begins rapidly (*acute* anemia) generally causes symptoms such as weakness or shortness of breath in children. Anemia that develops gradually and lasts for several months (*chronic* anemia) generally causes fewer symptoms.

Basic Types

Everybody is "expected" to have a certain number of red blood cells or amount of hemoglobin (red, iron-containing protein) in their blood. Anemia means either a lower-than-expected total number of red blood cells or a lower-than-expected amount of hemoglobin within the red blood cells. In some anemias there is a decrease in both hemoglobin and red blood cells.

Hemoglobin carries oxygen from the lungs to all the tissues of the body. It also carries the carbon dioxide (waste product) away from the tissues to the lungs so that it can be exhaled. As you can see, these functions are vital to your child's health.

Anemia can result from any of the following:

• Decrease in the production of red blood cells
• Decrease in hemoglobin formation

- Destruction of red blood cells
- Loss of blood such as from a hemorrhage or from intestinal bleeding.

Signs and Symptoms

It's important to be alert to signs of anemia in your child. Typical signs are: pallor of the skin and paleness of the lips, the inner lining of the eyelids, and the nail beds. Fatigue and irritability are also common symptoms. Severe anemia can also cause breathlessness, swelling of the hands and feet, and a rapid pulse.

Iron is normally found in a few essential tissues of the body, such as the blood and liver. When your child's blood is *iron-deficient*, he may have lowered resistance to infections. If this form of anemia persists for a long time, loss of appetite, and poor attention span may develop. There is also evidence that it may lead to a delay in physical and mental development.

The only reliable way to diagnose anemias is by having a *complete blood count* (referred to medically as a CBC). This is done by taking a blood sample from your child. A small amount of blood taken from your child's fingertip or toe may be enough to do the trick.

Common Causes

Young infants and children often become anemic because of malnutrition or because of dietary deficiencies, primarily lack of iron. If a mother doesn't ingest enough iron during pregnancy, both she and her newborn infant may develop anemia. If an infant drinks ordinary cow's milk (after six months of age) without taking iron-containing vitamins, iron-deficiency anemia often follows. The blood count will then show a hemoglobin level—the pigmented protein level within the red cells—lower than normal for the child's age.

This is the most common type of childhood anemia throughout the world.

Infections of various kinds can also cause anemia in childhood. Examples of these include intestinal parasites, hepatitis, infectious mononucleosis, and chronic intestinal diseases. Infections can either destroy red blood cells or suppress their normal production in the bone marrow.

Other Causes of Anemia

Familial or genetic anemias can appear in early infancy. Sickle-cell hemoglobin is a recessive trait (gene) found in about 10 percent of African Americans, who can carry the recessive trait without having the disease. Only one in 400 African Americans actually develop sickle-cell anemia, which is a very serious disease caused by the presence of two recessive sickle-cell genes (one from each parent).

Thalassemia is another type of anemia found in families of Asian or Mediterranean origin. This serious type of anemia, which is inherited, is characterized by abnormal hemoglobin.

When a child ingests certain chemicals or drugs, this can also lead to anemia. For example, the antibiotic *chloramphenicol*, commonly called chloromycetin, can suppress the bone marrow, causing aplastic anemia. The chemical benzene also has the same potential. This is another good reason to check labels and to ask your pediatrician about any known side effects when he prescribes a medication for your child.

Another cause of anemia in infants can be a blood group incompatibility between the mother and the fetus. The four blood groups are A, B, AB, O. In addition, blood can be Rh positive or negative. When the blood types are different and incompatible, the mother develops a sensitivity. Subsequent pregnancies of the mother may then result in her newborns developing *hemolytic anemias*, that is, anemias due to destruction of red blood cells. However, Rh incompatibility can easily be prevented if the mother receives an anti-Rh globulin injection shortly after her first delivery.

Preventive Measures

Infants and children on well-balanced formulas or diets will not develop nutritional anemias such as iron-deficiency anemia. As a rule, your infant should not be drinking cow's milk until he is about one year old. Cow's milk contains very little iron, and iron is always poorly absorbed from the intestine. The normal-weight, full-term infant on milk formula does not need any iron supplement before six months of age; the body stores iron received from the mother during the last stage of pregnancy, and this is adequate for growth in the early months despite the small amount of iron in the formula. Breast-fed infants also usually have enough iron to last until six months of age.

However, low birthweight (under 5½ pounds) and premature infants may require an iron supplement. These infants have less stored iron from the mother and will be growing at a fast rate. The smaller the birthweight, the greater the need for early iron supplementation. Your pediatrician can guide you in making this decision.

As a rule, toddlers and other children should regularly eat iron-containing foods. Iron-fortified cereal, eggs, red meat, and green and yellow vegetables are all rich in iron.

Alert!

To avoid a potentially serious medical problem, follow these rules:

1. Keep all iron medications out of the reach of small children. Such medications are very poisonous to children if taken in large amounts. *Lock cabinets and keep medication in childproof containers!*

2. Iron supplements can cause some children to become constipated. If you suspect this is happening, report the change you note to your doctor rather than abruptly discontinuing the iron supplement or vitamins he prescribed. (See Key 11 on constipation.)

What Parents Can Do

- Consult your doctor when you see signs and symptoms suggestive of anemia.
- Wait until your child is diagnosed with anemia *before* placing him on an iron supplement. Treatment for anemia should not begin until the exact type and cause of the anemia are determined by examination and laboratory tests.
- Wait to consult with your pediatrician before giving your child dietary supplements or vitamins.
- Ask the doctor about iron supplements or iron-fortified formula when your *full-term* infant reaches six months of age.
- Ask the doctor about iron supplements or iron-fortified formula when your *low birthweight* (under 5½ pounds) infant reaches one month of age.
- Inform the doctor about any family history of anemia when he checks the infant for the first time.
- When your child is no longer on milk formula or breast milk, make sure she maintains a well-balanced diet.

What the Doctor May Do

- Test for anemia by taking a blood sample and having a complete blood count (CBC).
- Recommend a formula with iron supplement or vitamins with iron for your infant.
- Review your child's diet to determine whether there is an adequate amount of iron-containing foods.
- Take a family history in order to rule out the possibility of genetic or familial anemias.

7

ASTHMA

Parents often become panicky when they hear the term "asthma," but the condition is usually not as serious as it sounds. People with asthma are prone to having asthma attacks, which can be mild or severe. What is an asthma attack? You can recognize one by a sudden wheezing or whistling sound with each breath. The sound is caused by a spasm of the smooth muscles that surround the airway tubes to the lungs. The spasm narrows these tubes (the bronchi and the smaller bronchioles) so that each outward breath produces a high-pitched sound known as a wheeze. In addition, the lining of the airway tubes becomes swollen and secretes a thick fluid called mucus.

How likely is your child to have asthma? Between 5 and 10 percent of children develop asthma in their early life—usually by five years of age. It usually begins as a sudden, acute attack, and it clears quickly with drugs called bronchodilators. Bronchodilators open up (or dilate) the airway tubes. The medication can be taken by mouth or by ventilator. School-aged children can be taught how to medicate themselves with a medicated inhaler when they feel an asthma attack coming on.

Some children have recurrent attacks of asthma (*chronic* asthma) later in childhood and in adulthood. Fortunately, most children who develop asthma before five years of age outgrow it by their adolescent years.

29

Signs and Symptoms

An asthmatic child wheezes or may have a persistent cough—especially at night—during an asthmatic attack. His chest wall may retract (pull inward) with each breath. Loud wheezing does not always mean that the attack is severe.

If the asthmatic attack is severe, your child may also have:

- Inability to speak more than a few words
- Short, rapid breathing
- Bluish coloration of lips and fingernails
- Agitation and anxiety

Vomiting may occur after bouts of coughing, and the child may feel more comfortable sitting upright. If left untreated, the attack may last for hours or days, and the child will become very fatigued.

In *chronic* asthma, the wheezing may be slight, but the coughing may be more noticeable at night. Cold air or exercise may trigger an attack in almost all children with this form of asthma.

Causes of Asthma

A variety of stress factors can trigger an asthmatic attack in a child whose body has a tendency (either inherited or acquired) to react this way. Stress factors can include substances in the environment, such as pollen and dust. Emotional distress is another factor that can set off an asthmatic attack. There are generally two different types of asthma: *allergic asthma* and *nonallergic asthma.*

Allergic asthma occurs in children who are sensitive to specific allergens such as pollens, dust, or molds. This is the most common form of asthma in children *over* five years. A few children with severe food allergies may also have allergic asthma attacks. (See family allergy history in Key 5 on allergies to foods.)

Nonallergic asthma occurs in children who have a wheezing reaction to other stimuli, such as respiratory infections, common colds, cold air, or emotional stress. This is the most common form of asthma in infants and preschool children, especially following a viral infection of the bronchi or bronchioles (see Key 8).

Other causes of asthma in some children are:

• Exercise
• Air pollutants, such as cigarette smoke or gasoline fumes
• Medications such as aspirin

Other Wheezing Conditions

There is an old saying among pediatricians: "All that wheezes is not asthma." However, other causes for wheezing can also be serious, and you should have your child checked out.

An infant under three months old may wheeze because of congenital birth malformations in her lungs, heart, or gastrointestinal tract.

A toddler may suddenly begin to wheeze after swallowing a foreign object (such as a coin) that blocks an air tube to the lung. It's rare for a coin to be stuck in the windpipe, but, if this happens, it can cause an acute breathing emergency. Usually the coin will lodge in a bronchial tube and cause only wheezing. In any case, an x-ray of the chest and a physical examination by the doctor are needed to help diagnose the sudden onset of wheezing.

What Parents Can Do

• If your infant or toddler suddenly begins to wheeze, she should be examined by the doctor immediately. If she has a known history of asthma, administer medication right away.

- Watch for signs of breathing trouble such as rapid breathing, chest retractions, blueness of the lips or fingernails, or difficulty speaking. If these occur, bring your child to the nearest emergency room and call your doctor.
- Other problems besides asthma (such as swallowing objects or having a respiratory infection) can cause wheezing. Your child must have a thorough physical examination to make a correct diagnosis.
- If your child is already diagnosed as having asthma, don't panic when you hear her wheeze. Loud wheezes often occur in mild attacks, and your emotional reaction may worsen the attack. Reassure her that she'll be all right and, if she's old enough to understand, explain what's happening.
- If your asthmatic child is taking medications but wheezing and coughing continue without relief, call the doctor again.
- If your asthmatic child vomits the oral medications, inform the doctor so that the medication can be given by another route, such as inhalation.
- If your child has allergic asthma, do all you can to keep his environment free of allergens. For example, you may need to keep him away from house dust, animal hair, or cigarette smoke.
- If exercise is a stressor that sets off asthma attacks, ask the doctor if you should inform the school about necessary restrictions in gym class. At home, work together to discover alternative, enjoyable activities.
- When your child is old enough to understand, teach her all about her asthmatic condition so that she can take proper care of herself, and when necessary, explain it to others.
- If emotional stress is a factor in triggering your child's asthma attacks, try to determine what is causing the upset and think of ways to reduce the stress.

What the Doctor May Do

- Take an x-ray of your child's chest and conduct a physical examination.
- Inquire about your child's reaction to various allergens and gather information to determine what triggered the wheezing.
- Prescribe medication in oral or inhaler form or give her an injection of an antiwheezing drug, if necessary.
- Help you develop a plan to remove allergens from the home.
- Refer your child to a pediatric allergist for skin testing and possible antiallergy injections throughout the year.

8

BRONCHITIS AND
BRONCHIOLITIS

Bronchitis is a common childhood illness. It is an inflammation or an infection of the large airway tubes, called bronchi, that lead to the lungs. Bronchiolitis is similar to bronchitis but occurs most frequently in infants under 18 months of age. Bronchiolitis is a respiratory illness of the smaller airways.

Bronchitis

Types of Bronchitis. There are three types of bronchitis: *acute infectious bronchitis*, *irritative bronchitis*, and *allergic bronchitis*.

The most common form of bronchitis is *acute infectious bronchitis*. This childhood illness is a lower respiratory infection that usually occurs in the cold months of the year after your child comes down with a common cold or other viral infection in the nose or throat (see Key 10 for more information on upper respiratory infections). Bacteria may complicate a common cold by infecting the nasal sinuses. When the infected mucus drips from the back of the nose ("postnasal drip"), bronchitis can result.

Another form of bronchitis is *irritative bronchitis*. This illness may occur in infants and children who are exposed to environmental dust, smog, and chemical fumes, or smoke. Tobacco smoke is the major irritant in homes of cigarette-smoking parents.

The third form of bronchitis is *allergic bronchitis* (see Key 7 on asthma), which can produce coughing without wheezing. This type of bronchitis may occur when an allergic or asthmatic child enters an environment and inhales an allergen to which she is sensitive.

Symptoms of Infectious Bronchitis. After the symptoms of a common cold (runny nose, sneezing, chills, and slight fever) appear, a dry cough may begin. In a day or more, the coughing increases and sounds wet and deep. Occasional thick, yellow, or white mucus may be expelled with some coughs.

Spells of repeated coughs may develop later. Breathing may become noisy and be accompanied by the rattling sounds of mucus in the bronchi or by wheezing.

When should you call the doctor? Call if your child becomes irritable or restless or if he has trouble sleeping and eating. Call the doctor immediately if you see your child having difficulty breathing and you notice the chest pulling inward below the ribs or above the breastbone.

In bronchitis, a low-grade fever (101° to 102°F) may continue for a few days, but the cough may linger and then gradually fade over the next few weeks. Although acute bronchitis is usually a mild illness, it can lead to complications such as pneumonia. (For this reason, it is important to seek medical attention in the early stages.)

Attacks of acute bronchitis that last for months or that recur often over many years are termed *chronic bronchitis*. This condition is usually associated with allergies, chronic lung disease, or chronic sinusitis, because these long-term illnesses tend to have repeated episodes that trigger inflammation in the bronchial tubes.

Bronchiolitis in Young Infants

The illness of infants called bronchiolitis involves an infection of the small airway tubes, called bronchioles. It is caused by respiratory viruses.

By the time infants become toddlers, between 10 and 15 percent of them will have had bronchiolitis. About half of these will develop asthma at an older age. Interestingly, the reason for this relationship is still unknown.

Causes of Bronchiolitis. A young infant or toddler usually catches respiratory viruses from family members or from infected infants or children he has come in contact with. These viral infections mostly occur in the colder months of the year (fall through early spring). Nose and throat secretions (from sneezing, coughing, and talking) spread the virus particles, which float in the air as microscopic droplets. Other children in the room inhale these particles and, after one to 10 days of incubation in their nose and throat, they exhibit symptoms.

Inflammation of the lining cells also causes swelling and secretions of mucus. As a result, the bronchioles become plugged with mucus and dead cells, and it becomes difficult for air to enter or leave these airways.

Symptoms of Bronchiolitis. During the first couple of days, if your infant is infected, he may have sneezing, runny nose, coughing, wheezing, and low-grade fever ($101°$ to $102°F$). As the illness progresses, his breathing will become rapid and strained because fresh air (oxygen) can't reach his lungs and stale air (carbon dioxide) is trapped in his blocked lung airways. At that point, your infant might become very tired and, if his case is severe, he may be unable to drink adequate amounts of fluids. This can be a frightening experience for parents. Even though it may be difficult, try to *prevent dehydration* by offering small amounts of clear liquids to your child every half hour.

In infants, bronchiolitis usually subsides in about five days. Older children infected with the same respiratory viruses usually come down with symptoms of a common cold only. That is because most older children when they were younger had prior infections with the same viruses and over time developed a partial immunity.

Respiratory Distress
Symptoms of respiratory distress include:

- Fast breathing
- Dilating nostrils
- Pulling inward of chest wall (between ribs, below ribs, or above breastbone)
- Grunting or wheezing with each breath
- Bluish discoloration of lips or fingernails *(NOTE: This is an acute emergency.)*

The presence of any of these signs is a red flag for parents. Contact your doctor immediately or take your child to the emergency room as soon as possible. In a small percentage of cases, hospitalization may be necessary for oxygen, drug therapy, and intravenous fluids.

What Parents Can Do
- Keep in mind that not all "cold" symptoms are due to common colds. Most respiratory viruses begin as colds but become worse instead of better in a few days.
- Have your infant or child examined by a doctor if a "cold" doesn't improve after five days or if she has breathing distress (see above signs) at any time.
- Keep a close watch on your infant or child—day and night—if she develops a deep cough or noisy breathing (either wheezing or grunting).

- As much as possible, limit the exposure of infants and toddlers to indoor crowds of adults and children during the cold months. Day-care environments and play groups are risks during these months but it's a trade-off and, for many people, a necessity.
- Avoid family friends and relatives who have colds or respiratory infections. Your infants and toddlers should not be in close contact with, or even in the same room with, people who are infected.

What the Doctor May Do

- Conduct a thorough medical examination, including listening to your child's lungs.
- Possibly take a chest x-ray.
- Prescribe antibiotics if she diagnoses your child as having a respiratory infection.
- Recommend that you place a cool-air vaporizer in your child's room.
- Prescribe a cough medicine or decongestant.

9

CHICKENPOX

C hickenpox, an itchy, blister-forming rash that can cover much of the body, is, next to the common cold, probably the most easily spread (contagious) disease of childhood. In the average U.S. community, 90 percent or more of children acquire this disease by the time they are 15 years old. Most cases occur between five and 10 years of age, usually in the winter and spring months.

Even though chickenpox is highly contagious, it is usually not cause for alarm. Complications are rare in children and are more likely to occur in adults and newborn infants whose mothers never had the disease.

Cause

Chickenpox is caused by a virus in the *herpes* family called the *varicella-zoster* (V-Z) virus. After your child has the disease, the virus will remain dormant (quiet) in the nerves near the spinal cord for the rest of his life. Immunity is life-long, so that once he has had chickenpox, you don't have to worry that he's going to catch it again. However, there are some rare exceptions. My younger son, for example, had chicken pox twice! Older adults—usually over the age of 50—may begin to lose some of their immunity. The same dormant virus can then be reactivated to cause *shingles*, a painful skin disease.

How the Virus Spreads

Your child can easily catch the virus by being in close contact with another child who has the disease. The virus particles of the sick child are in the blisters (also called *vesicles*) of the skin rash and in the nose and throat. The particles enter the room air as microscopic droplets from nose and throat secretions or from discharges that come from opened skin blisters. Once your child inhales the room air, touches the skin blisters, or touches clothing that was soiled with these discharges, he can become infected with the virus. A child can also catch chickenpox from a person with shingles.

Since chickenpox is spread so readily by airborne droplets, it is extremely difficult to completely isolate the disease. Keeping a child with chickenpox in his room won't really be effective in reducing the risk to other family members. The virus particles can float throughout the house and even through cracks in the door. Other susceptible children or adults in the same household have at least a 90 percent chance of catching the virus, even if physically separated from the ill child.

Chickenpox is contagious from two days before the rash begins until five days after the rash first appears. This means there is about a seven-day span in which the disease can spread.

Symptoms

There is an incubation period for chickenpox, which means that there is a gap between the time your child is exposed to the virus and the time symptoms first appear. Usually two to three weeks after exposure to the virus, a child who is infected will come down with a low fever and loss of appetite. By the next day, a rash may erupt on the trunk or anywhere on the body, including the scalp, mouth, or eyes. The rash begins as small, red pimples. In a few hours these change to "teardrop" blisters (or vesicles), which are very itchy. New batches of these vesicles keep cropping up over the next three or four days, while the old ones open up, become crusted, and scab. Some children develop a couple of hundred lesions, and some, less than a dozen.

Regardless of the number, the blisters cause discomfort and can make your child irritable. In order to relieve the itching, ask your doctor to prescribe an antihistamine and to recommend a soothing lotion for the skin. Parents often worry that the scars from the chickenpox will become permanent. Rest assured that the pink marks will be gone in a few weeks.

Besides the blisters, some children develop high fever (104°F or more). It is very important that you do not give aspirin to relieve the fever. When aspirin is given to children with chickenpox or influenza (the "flu"), they can suddenly develop *Reye syndrome*, which is a rare and serious or fatal condition affecting the liver and brain. Symptoms include bouts of vomiting every couple of hours followed by coma or seizures. In order to reduce the risk of Reye syndrome, it is best to use acetaminophen (such as Tylenol® or its equivalent) instead of aspirin for fever control. When a child with chickenpox has fever, the fever usually doesn't last very long.

Complications

Although it is usually a benign illness, complications are possible. The most common problem is secondary skin infection due to scratching of the skin. If deep skin infections do occur, permanent scars may result. The best preventive measures are:

1. Relieve the itching with medications and lotions prescribed by the doctor.
2. Cut your child's fingernails short.
3. Make sure your child's skin and nails are clean.

Keep in mind that the skin usually does not become infected and that, in most cases, the marks soon go away.

41

Complications involving the blood or nervous system are possible, but these are very rare in healthy children. Drowsiness or frequent vomiting after two or three days of the illness should be quickly reported to the doctor for her evaluation.

Early Exposure to Chickenpox

Newborn infants (except very premature babies) whose mothers are immune to chickenpox will be immune to the disease for the first few months of life. But when chickenpox occurs during the first 10 days of a baby's life and the mother is not immune to it, a severe or fatal case can result. About 50 percent of newborns will contract the disease if the mother develops chickenpox within the five-day period before and the two-day period after delivery.

Congenital Varicella

If chickenpox occurs in the first few months of pregnancy, there is a chance that the mother may pass this disease to her baby in the womb. This is called *congenital varicella*, and about 2 percent of the time it causes fetal abnormalities affecting the limbs, brain, or eyes. Pregnant women who are exposed to the disease during the early months of pregnancy should make a strong effort to find out if they had chickenpox when younger. If they are in doubt, they can take a blood test to determine whether they have the immunity. They should discuss with their doctor the need for antibody testing. About 90 percent of the time, the test shows immunity even if there is no history of the disease. The main purpose of the immunity test is to provide reassurance to about 90 percent of the exposed women who have no known history of chickenpox. The fetus in the womb is completely protected against the disease if the mother shows immunity.

Prevention

Modified chickenpox vaccines have recently been developed, and many thousands of children in Japan have already received one type of the vaccine. It has provided good protection without serious side effects. For the past few years, there have been clinical trials of a similar vaccine in the United States, and it may be licensed for general use in 1993. Meanwhile, don't expose your child to a case of chickenpox deliberately to give him immunity.

At the present time, high-risk children (such as those receiving corticosteroids or chemotherapy) who have never had chickenpox can receive an injection of the varicella antibody (VZIG) within four days after first contact with a known case. This injection either prevents the chicken pox completely or ensures a very mild case.

The chickenpox antibody (VZIG) can also be given to pregnant women who do not have immunity to chickenpox and who are exposed to the disease in the first half of pregnancy. It should also be given within four days to any newborn infant whose mother came down with chickenpox within five days before delivery or within two days after delivery. Small premature infants who are exposed to the virus during their first few weeks in the hospital nursery may also be candidates for VZIG within four days of their contact with the disease.

What Parents Can Do

- Do your best to avoid exposing your infant or child to chickenpox. If he hasn't had the disease, don't bring him to a home where there is a person with chickenpox or shingles—even if that person is in a separate, closed room elsewhere in the house.
- If your child has itchy, red pimples with tiny blisters at the center, call the doctor. Ask her when she can examine your child at the office without having him sit in the waiting room where he may expose other children to the disease.

- If the doctor makes the diagnosis of chickenpox, keep a written record of the date and the doctor's name. Essential medical records containing the history of the diseases and immunizations for each of your children should be kept in a safe place for future reference when they become adults. (See Appendix B.)
- Ask the doctor to prescribe medication for the itching and to recommend a skin lotion.
- To safeguard against skin infections, cut your child's fingernails short. Keep his fingernails and skin clean.
- Use acetaminophen (such as Tylenol®) if your child has fever. *Don't ever give aspirin to your child if he has chickenpox (or the "flu")*.

What the Doctor May Do

- Inquire whether other members of the household ever had chickenpox.
- Possibly administer an injection of the chickenpox antibody, medically referred to as VZIG, to a chicken pox-exposed pregnant women who does not show immunity to chickenpox on a blood test, a newborn infant whose mother came down with chickenpox around the time of the delivery, or a premature baby who has been exposed to the virus. (Unfortunately, it has not been proven that the VZIG injection prevents chickenpox in all cases.)
- Prescribe medication for the itching that causes discomfort to your child.
- Recommend acetaminophen or another nonaspirin equivalent to relieve fever and discomfort.

10

COMMON COLDS AND
UPPER RESPIRATORY
INFECTIONS

O f all the illnesses your child may have, you will probably become the most familiar with upper respiratory
infections such as the "common cold" and the "flu."
Your young school-aged child will catch a few colds and
upper respiratory infections (URIs) each year until she reaches adolescence. Your preschool child who attends a day-care
center or a nursery school or who has an older sibling in elementary school is more likely to come down with these infections than a child who doesn't have these risk factors. But the
first year in any children's group setting always results in
many URIs, which your preschooler can handle without too
much trouble.

Upper respiratory infections are infections that involve
the nose, throat, sinuses (hollow spaces connected to the
nasal passages), larynx (voice box), trachea (windpipe), or
upper bronchi (large airways to the lungs). These infections
are highly contagious and are the most common infections in
both children and adults. People can catch upper respiratory
infections any time of the year, but they are especially common during the cold-weather months. If your child has this
type of infection, her symptoms will probably last several
days and subside without antibiotic treatment and without

complications. However, the symptoms can cause discomfort, and she may be especially irritable and demanding during this time.

Causes

There are more than 100 different types of viruses that cause upper respiratory infection in infants and children. The influenza virus ("flu") causes URIs with fever, fatigue, and generalized body aches that last for several days. There are many common cold viruses that cause URIs, and it's difficult to tell them apart without special cultures for viruses. Some infectious disease experts believe that the cause of over half the cases of common colds is still unknown.

Contrary to folk wisdom or what your mother might have told you, drafts and chills do not bring on colds or upper respiratory infections. Enlarged tonsils and adenoids do not make a child more susceptible to colds or URIs. However, if your child is fatigued or under emotional stress or is having a nasal allergy attack, she can have lower resistance to these viruses. If she then comes in close contact with someone who has a cold or URI, she can more easily catch it.

After a cold or other upper respiratory infection begins, bacteria such as staphylococcus, which normally live peacefully in the nose of many children, can occasionally complicate the condition and cause a secondary infection of the sinuses (sinusitis), middle ear (otitis media), or bronchi (bronchitis).

Symptoms

After an *incubation period* (the time between the contact with the infectious agent and the first sign of illness) that lasts from one to five days, sneezing and runny nose symptoms begin. Unlike infants and toddlers, children around four or five years old often complain of a sore throat and chilliness. Unlike older children, infants and toddlers can become very irritable and run a low-grade fever (100° to 102°F), especially in the evening. The sneezing and clear, watery secretions from the nose gradually decrease, and after a couple of days the nose becomes clogged with thick, yellow, or green mucus. Coughing usually begins, especially during the night, due to postnasal drip. If your child has laryngitis, her cry or voice will sound hoarse. If your child's cough continues for a week without improvement or if her cough begins to sound either hoarse ("croupy") or "deep in chest," have the doctor examine her.

If your child is feverish, keep her indoors. If her temperature rises to 103° to 104°F or if her low-grade fever continues for two or three days, it is a good idea to call her doctor.

If your infant has a congested nose, it may be difficult to feed her. This is because infants have not yet learned to breathe through their mouth when necessary. To help relieve congestion, use nose drops and a nasal aspirator, which is a nose suction bulb. Complications following upper respiratory infections (such as bronchitis) happen more often in small infants than in toddlers or school-aged children.

Spread of the Viruses

Upper respiratory infections are most contagious during the 24 hours before symptoms begin and during the five days after symptoms begin. You have to be in close contact with a person who has a cold before you catch it. Perhaps that's why mothers usually catch colds from their children more often than fathers do.

These viral infections spread from person to person in several ways:

• By direct contact with nose or throat secretions (mucus) of an infected person

KEYS TO CHILDHOOD ILLNESSES

- By inhaling airborne droplets of these secretions
- By touching articles (such as toys, clothing, silverware) soiled by infected secretions and then touching your nose or eyes with your fingers
- By touching the hands of an infected person and then wiping your nose and eyes with your fingers

Resistance to Colds and Upper Respiratory Infections

People of all ages—including newborns and young infants—are susceptible to viral infections. Having a cold or URI leads to antibody formation in about two weeks. But these antibodies don't last long, and resistance to future infection by these viruses is short-lived. Another reason that resistance is poor is that a very large number and variety of these virus groups can cause the same symptoms, and each group has many subtypes within it. For example, a child who has experienced an infection with *adenovirus* type 7 will not develop any immunity at all to *adenovirus* type 14.

Prevention

Vaccines against these viruses have not been formulated because there are so many groups and subtypes. Large doses of vitamin C do not increase the resistance to colds or URIs, despite popular claims.

The best prevention is to have your child avoid close contact—especially indoors—with an adult or child who has a URI. This generally means avoiding close contact during the early stage (the first five days) of the person's illness. Politely suggest to an ill person that he cover his mouth when coughing and cover his nose before sneezing. Teach your children these same preventive measures when they're two or three years old.

If you are ill and caring for a newborn or young infant, you can wear a paper or cloth mask over your nose and mouth. You should also wash your hands before handling your children or before touching their toys, clothing, or food. Needless to say, an infected adult or child should not kiss your child's hands, face, or head. Whenever practical, opening windows and "airing out" rooms for at least one hour will reduce the number of virus droplets floating in the indoor air.

Discourage any friends and relatives (and their children) who have upper respiratory infections from visiting you and your children at home. Although it may be inconvenient, it's best to postpone your visits to them and their children when you and your children have URIs.

What Parents Can Do

- When your child has a URI, you can ease her discomfort by using nose drops, a nasal aspirator (nose suction bulb), and a decongestant. Place a vaporizer in the room when she sleeps.
- During the cold and "flu" months, try to avoid bringing your infant or toddler to crowded indoor areas such as supermarkets, house parties, or restaurants. The reality is that this is often difficult to arrange, but do your best. Preschoolers (those three to five years old) can handle URIs better than younger children.
- Day-care facilities, nursery schools, and play groups are common places for URIs to spread from one child to another. If your child has symptoms such as fatigue, fever (of any kind), or a constant cough, keep her at home.
- Whenever possible and practical, avoid close contacts—especially indoors—between your young children and any adult or child who has early URI symptoms like runny nose, sneezing, or coughing. If possible, try to prevent your child from playing with a sick child's toys unless they can be washed first.

- Discourage an ill adult or child from touching the skin or clothing of your child. Encourage handwashing and wearing of a mask when they visit.

- Call the doctor or bring your child in for an examination if a low-grade fever goes beyond two to three days or if a high fever (103° to 104°F) occurs at any time.

- Call the doctor if your child's coughing lasts more than five days or if it begins to sound hoarse ("croupy") or "deep in chest."

- Children with chronic diseases such as heart or lung conditions generally benefit from immunization with "flu" injections at the beginning of the cold season. However, if your child is healthy, she can resist complications of upper respiratory infections, and the "flu" injection is not necessary.

What the Doctor May Do

- Take a nose and throat culture.
- Take a blood sample to get a complete blood count.
- Take a chest x-ray if your child's cough and fever continue for several days.
- Possibly prescribe an antibiotic (to prevent or treat complications).
- Advise you to use acetaminophen (such as Tylenol®) for fever.
- Recommend that your child remain indoors until she no longer has a fever.
- Advise you to use nose drops, a vaporizer, or a nasal aspirator in order to relieve your child's discomfort.
- Advise you to place your child on a regular diet (if there's no decrease in appetite) and to increase her fluid intake.

11

CONSTIPATION

A n infant or child has *constipation* when he passes dry, hard stools (feces) or when he has infrequent bowel movements. It is important to keep in mind that there is a wide range of "normal" with regard to the frequency of bowel movements and the consistency of the stool. Most infants pass stool about once daily, but some regularly pass as many as five stools each day. On the other hand, some healthy infants may pass one every third day. It is usual for older children to have a bowel movement once daily, but there can be a normal range from two or three each day in some children to one every three or four days in other children. However, once your infant or child establishes his "regularity" habit (what is normal for him), you should be alert to those days when the pattern changes or when the stools become too hard or painful for him to pass.

Causes

When constipation occurs, there may occasionally be a physical cause such as the following:

- Decreased contraction of the intestinal wall muscles (called peristalsis)
- Weakness of the abdominal muscles
- A blockage within the large intestine or rectum

These conditions usually result from congenital (birth) defects, formula or dietary changes, drug side effects, or inflammatory conditions of the rectum.

The most frequent cause of constipation in toddlers and young children is voluntary withholding of stool (called *functional* constipation). Often there is a familial tendency toward this problem, and it usually begins with toilet training. For example, forcible or overly strict "potty" training may cause resistance and voluntary withholding of stools. Feelings of shame or embarrassment over the stool can also cause voluntary withholding.

Why does constipation occur? When the stool remains longer in the large intestine and rectum, water is reabsorbed by the body and the stool becomes dry and hard. When a movement does occur, it can be painful. From then on, fear of defecation may cause more voluntary withholding by the child. A vicious cycle develops in which the child's efforts to avoid the pain by withholding the stool can actually worsen the constipation. In addition, the continuously withheld stool increases in size and hardness and gradually stretches the wall of the colon. The wall then loses its muscular strength, and the urge to "move" is thereby lessened.

Symptoms

The most noticeable sign of constipation is hard, dry stools that are painful or that take a long time to pass. At times, a child who has chronic constipation may appear to pass watery stools that resemble diarrhea. But this can be deceptive, for it may indicate "overflow diarrhea," which occurs when a very large stool remains in the rectum and some fecal fluid from the intestine above it leaks around it. Often this fluid causes soiling of the underwear.

Abdominal pains and the release of gas by the rectum can be part of a constipation problem. Passing a large stool will usually relieve these symptoms. If your infant or young child shows signs of straining more than usual during a bowel movement, check to see if the stool appears hard and compact. (See Key 3 for more on abdominal pains.)

Complications

If the problem is unrelieved and becomes long-lasting, some difficulties can arise. One of these is known as *anal fissures*, which are small ulcers or cracks in the skin around the anal opening. They are painful and can cause blood streaks on the stool or underwear. A more serious abnormality following a prolonged constipation is *fecal impaction*. In this condition, the stool in the rectum becomes so large and hard that it resembles solid putty, and it can completely block the lower intestine. *Urinary tract infections* can also result from severe chronic constipation that can block the urinary bladder. (See Key 33 for more on urinary tract infections.)

When a child over four years of age loses bowel control and soils day or night, the disease is called *encopresis*. Encopresis is not a common occurrence, as it is found in only 1 percent of school-aged children. This problem can develop in children who have either intermittent constipation or regular bowel movements that are incomplete. Many of these children have lost their normal sensation ("urge") to defecate and have therefore lost some bowel control.

Encopresis can cause stress in the family, and there is a tendency for parents to get involved in a power struggle with their child over the soiling. Try to avoid acting on your anger, as this will only compound the problem. Instead, have your pediatrician evaluate your child to determine what is causing the encopresis. Sometimes severe psychological stress in the child or the family leads to encopresis.

If the pediatrician does not find a physical cause, consult with a psychologist, who can evaluate any emotional causes and advise you about proper behavioral management of the encopresis. (Also see Key 15.)

In the case of *chronic constipation*, that is, constipation that continues or recurs over several months, rely on your pediatrician to make a proper diagnosis and help you manage any complications.

Prevention

You should begin a daily toilet training program for your toddler when she is around two years of age. Before that time, it is unlikely that she will have the physical control to be successful. Proceed gradually, and use a lot of support and praise. Having a critical attitude or pressuring your child may only serve to inhibit her and frustrate you both.

It is realistic to expect that there will be "accidents," especially in the early stages of toilet training and in places where the child is not familiar. Successful toilet-training takes time, and each child is different. Good training and an accepting outlook will help your child develop a regular, daily bowel habit and feel proud of her achievement.

You may want to consult with your pediatrician about the steps you should take in setting up a toilet-training program for your child. There are also several helpful books written for children to introduce them to the idea of toilet training.

What Parents Can Do

- Gradually begin toilet training when your child is about two years old. Ask your doctor if she feels this is the right time for your child and about the best way to proceed.
- Avoid overly strict toilet training in which you use punishment or express anger and disappointment. Praise, support, and encouragement will help your child learn this new behavior and feel good about himself.
- Keep a daily check on your child's bowel movements. Make a mental note of the consistency, size, and frequency. If she

has a daily movement as a habit, call the doctor if she passes no stool in three days or if there is any sign of blood or pain during any movement.

- Notify the doctor if you see stool-soiling of the underwear in your child over four years old.
- Be alert for formula or dietary changes that harden the stool. Ask the doctor for advice.
- Include high-fiber foods (such as prunes, apricots, or peaches) in your child's daily diet if she is over one year old. Avoid bananas, apples, and rice.
- Avoid using laxatives, enemas, or suppositories without the doctor's advice. If you're not careful, they can become habit-forming.

What the Doctor May Do

- Ask how often your child usually has a bowel movement and about the consistency of the stool.
- Ask whether your child is experiencing pain in passing the stool or if there is any blood in the stool.
- Inquire about your child's intake of foods and liquids.
- Conduct a thorough physical examination.
- In the case of regular soiling in a child over four years of age, inquire about any stress factors in your child's life.

12

CROUP

If your child develops a hoarse voice along with a cough that sounds like a barking dog or a seal, he probably has croup. *Croup* is a respiratory illness caused by an inflammation of the vocal cords (also known as larynx) or an inflammation of the windpipe and airway tubes (trachea and bronchi). A severe form of croup (usually in children two to four years old) is due to *epiglottitis* (inflammation of the lid that covers the vocal cords). The croupy sound your child makes can be alarming to many parents. Call the doctor immediately for advice.

Causes

There are three different types of croup: *viral, bacterial,* and *spasmodic.*

The most common type of croup is *viral croup*. This is caused by a viral infection that invades the voice box (larynx) and the windpipe (trachea) of children six months to six years old during the fall and winter. Of the many viruses that cause acute respiratory infections, the *parainfluenza* virus is the one most responsible for croup. But many other respiratory viruses—including the *common cold* virus—can also do it.

The dangerous *bacterial croup*, epiglottitis, is almost always due to bacterium known as *H. influenzae, type b*. In these cases, the swelling of the epiglottis can result in a serious block to breathing.

The cause of *spasmodic croup* is not well understood. However, it may be an allergic reaction and tends to recur in some children.

Sometimes other factors can cause a condition that seems like croup. Although rare, a food or pollen allergy can cause swelling of the epiglottis and a croupy condition. A swallowed foreign object such as a coin or toy can be caught in the vocal cords and cause a sound like croup as a result of infection.

Symptoms

Cold symptoms such as runny nose, cough, and fever generally arrive before the croup. As the infection travels down to the lining of the vocal cords and upper airways, more secretions occur, and swelling of these tissues begins. A hoarse voice may follow, and the cough becomes "barklike." These symptoms usually worsen at night, and the illness continues for three or four days.

In some cases, the tissues swell a great deal, and breathing becomes difficult. When this occurs, a child's breathing can sound like a whistle. The lower ribs and the soft tissues of the neck may retract, or begin to pull inward, with each breath as air intake is blocked. As this occurs, the child may have rapid breathing, restlessness, and sweating. If these symptoms progress, bluish discoloration (medically known as cyanosis) of the lips and nail beds may occur. Look for these symptoms, as they indicate that your child needs to be seen immediately by your doctor or taken to the nearest emergency room.

Bacterial croup (caused by the *H. influenzae* bacterium) begins quickly and progresses rapidly. In addition to high fever, your child may have trouble breathing and difficulty swallowing. The voice may not become hoarse, but it may sound "muffled." If the child coughs, the cough may not sound like a bark. While struggling for air, the child may drool and wheeze. Extreme restlessness, exhaustion, chest contractions, and cyanosis may follow. At this stage, you have a true medical emergency. Immediately bring your child to the nearest emergency room.

Spasmodic croup usually awakens the child suddenly during the night even though he did not have any symptoms during that day. The hoarse voice and barking cough disappear the next day but come back during the next two or three nights. Generally, spasmodic croup does not become severe, but some children have repeated episodes up to six years of age.

Prevention

For *viral croup*, the major preventive measure is the avoidance of close contacts with children or adults who have upper respiratory infections or colds (see Key 10 for more information on prevention).

To prevent *bacterial croup*, several vaccines are now available. Some of them can be given to infants as young as two months old and children as old as five years. Depending on the age of the child, the number of doses (injections) ranges from one to four. These vaccines have few side effects and protect your infant or child against the type of meningitis caused by the same *H. influenzae* bacterium.

If a child comes down with bacterial croup and there is another child in the same household younger than four years, special preventive measures are recommended for all family members regardless of their ages. This includes all children, even if they have received the vaccine previously. In this situation, a special antibiotic (rifampin) is given for four days to all members of the household.

What Parents Can Do

- If your child develops a hoarse voice and a barking cough, contact the doctor as soon as possible.
- If your child develops croup, remain near the child at home day and night, and watch for any of these signs that the condition is worsening:
  - Difficult, fast breathing
  - Whistling breath sounds
  - Retractions in neck or below ribs
  - Restlessness and exhaustion
  - Cyanosis (bluish discoloration) of lips or nail beds.
- Immediately bring your child to your doctor or to the nearest hospital emergency room if she shows any of the signs listed above.
- For temporary relief of the barklike cough, place your child in a steam-filled room or in a room that has a cold-air humidifier.

What the Doctor May Do

- Listen to your child's chest.
- Examine your child's throat to see if the *epiglottis* is red and swollen. (This is usually a sign of bacterial croup.) This type of exam may be done in her office or in the hospital emergency room.
- Prescribe an antibiotic if your child is diagnosed as having *bacterial croup.*
- Hospitalize your child immediately for treatment.

13

DIARRHEA

When your child has diarrhea, there has been a change in the frequency and the consistency of her stool. She is having frequent bowel movements, and they are more loose or watery than usual. Each child is different, and it's important for you to know your child's routine (how often she usually has a bowel movement, as well as what the usual consistency of her stool is like).

Diarrhea is a common occurrence in childhood. The average child probably has one or two episodes of diarrhea each year, but an occasional loose movement on some days doesn't mean diarrhea. When an infant passes more than six to eight loose stools in a day, she has diarrhea. (Some breast-fed infants normally pass up to 12 soft stools a day for a couple of months after birth, but these are not watery.) When a child over one year of age has more than three to four loose stools in a day, she has diarrhea.

Causes

Diarrhea can be acute or chronic. *Acute diarrhea* lasts for a period of a few days, whereas *chronic diarrhea* is continuous or intermittent over a period of weeks or months.

Acute diarrhea can be caused by a viral infection, a bacterial infection, or food poisoning or can be a reaction to antibiotics. These conditions interfere with the normal functioning of the intestines in one of two ways. The intestines may absorb less water back into the bloodstream, or there may be increased secretion of water and chemical substances (electrolytes) from the inner lining cells of the intestines. In either case, the result is the presence of too much water in the stool (feces).

In infants and children, the most common cause of acute diarrhea is *gastroenteritis* (inflammation of the lining of the intestinal tract). This condition usually results from infections by certain types of viruses known as enteroviruses.

Another less common cause is harmful bacteria that may be spread to children in some contaminated foods or water. Some examples of these bacteria are: *salmonella, E. coli,* and *campylobacter*. Some intestinal bacteria can also be spread directly from person to person (fingers to objects to mouth).

Diarrhea can also follow food poisoning by chemicals or toxins that contaminate some foods. For example, toxins in certain wild mushrooms and certain fishes can cause diarrhea and other symptoms of illness. (See Key 16 on food poisoning.)

Occasionally, diarrhea in infants and toddlers is caused by a bacterial infection that is not in the intestinal tract. For instance, a middle ear infection or pneumonia in very young children can produce diarrhea in addition to other symptoms of the infections.

Many antibiotics can cause diarrhea in children of any age if these medications are taken for a long period of time. You should notify the doctor who prescribed the antibiotic if this side effect develops during the treatment of an infection.

Food or milk allergies can also induce diarrhea in some infants and children. A large intake of high-fiber foods such as certain fruits and vegetables can be another cause. Some toddlers who drink large amounts of fruit juices or heavily sweetened drinks can develop diarrhea.

Chronic diarrhea means that the condition continues or recurs over weeks or months. In these cases, some chronic intestinal diseases, such as celiac disease, irritable bowel (colon), and stomach enzyme deficiency, and milk sugar (lactose) intolerance have to be ruled out by the doctor and laboratory testing. Special management of these diseases is required.

Symptoms

Although caused by the same agents, the symptoms of a disease can vary from child to child. Mild cases of diarrhea show only a small change in the usual pattern of consistency and frequency of the bowel movements. Severe cases have green, watery stools mixed with mucus, blood, or pus every hour or two. Vomiting and fever usually accompany diarrhea caused by viral gastronenteritis. Abdominal cramps can occur before and during the movements. In severe diarrhea, there may be a high fever, listlessness, and loss of appetite. When you see these symptoms in your child, contact the doctor for immediate advice.

Dehydration

The combination of diarrhea and vomiting can be serious because it dehydrates the child. That means the body loses large amounts of water and chemicals (electolytes) that are essential for the normal functioning of all body cells. Dehydration can develop more quickly in infants and toddlers because of their small bodies. To prevent dehydration, ask the pediatrician whether she recommends that you give your child an electrolyte solution (such as Pedialyte®). This is a liquid that your child can either drink or take in his bottle.

When a child gets dehydrated, it is a serious matter. Call the doctor as soon as possible if you notice any of the following signs:

- No urination for six hours (child) or wetting less than six diapers in 24 hours (infant)
- Dry lips, tongue, or mouth
- Irritability and restlessness
- Increased sleepiness
- Fever rising to 104°F or higher

When severe dehydration develops, hospitalization is often necessary to allow for intravenous water and electrolyte replacement.

What Parents Can Do

- Call the doctor if your child has the following:
  - Mild diarrhea plus fever for more than 24 hours
  - Severe diarrhea (watery stools every hour or two)
  - Blood or mucus in her stool
  - Severe abdominal pain with diarrhea
  - Signs of dehydration (see above section)
  - Mild diarrhea without fever that continues for one week.
- Avoid using antidiarrheal medications sold over the counter until you check with your doctor. Some of these medications do more harm than good.
- Avoid prolonged use of antibiotics unless advised to do so by the doctor.
- Put your child on a bland diet including gelatin dessert, tea, toast, rice, apples, and bananas. Try rice cereal with an infant (some are prepared with bananas).
- Avoid feeding your child any fruits or fruit juices (except for apples and bananas).

What the Doctor May Do

- Ask when the diarrhea started, whether there has been any change in your child's diet, and what the frequency and consistency of the stool are like.

- Inquire whether any other members of the household are having these symptoms.
- Prescribe medication for the diarrhea.
- Recommend an electrolyte solution (such as Pedialyte®) to prevent dehydration.
- Watch closely for signs of dehydration if your child has both vomiting and diarrhea.
- Advise a special diet and limited activities for several days.
- Take a stool sample for bacterial culture.
- Hospitalize your child for intravenous fluid therapy if dehydration becomes severe.

14

EAR INFECTIONS

E ar infections are fairly common in infants and young children. The symptoms may be painful, but they are easy to treat. Complications caused by ear infections can usually be prevented with early and adequate treatment.

There are two types of ear infections: middle ear infections and external ear infections. The only way to determine which type of infection your child has is by physical examination.

Middle Ear Infection

The middle ear is a tiny box deep in the ear canal behind the eardrum. Infections of the middle ear occur most often between four months and five years of age. They usually occur after a cold or upper respiratory infection (URI). Infants and preschool children can easily catch colds and upper respiratory infections that lead to middle ear infections. These infections develop most often in the cold months of winter and spring. By three years of age, about 75 percent of children have had one or more bouts of this illness. This means that the majority of young children have ear infections at one time or another and that some children frequently have earaches.

Causes. Bacteria and viruses in the nose or throat can easily travel to the middle ear through the eustachian tube, which connects the back of the nasal cavity to the middle ear. In infants and toddlers, this tube is short and wide and runs horizontally. Infected fluid can quickly spread from the nose to the middle ear. The eustachian tube can become blocked by a nose or throat infection or by large adenoids. (See Key 4 on adenoid and tonsil problems.) If this occurs, the infection cannot drain itself from the middle ear. Instead, the bacteria or viruses remain in the middle ear and multiply. Infected fluid (pus) then accumulates, and the eardrum bulges and may open. As this occurs, discharge leaks into the outer ear canal.

If your young child gets lots of ear infections, it's likely that this problem will improve as he gets older. By school age, the shape of the eustachian tube changes, and ear infections occur less frequently.

Allergies like hay fever can sometimes cause an inflammation of the middle ear that resembles a middle ear infection, but this is not the same thing as an infection.

Symptoms. Ear pain is the chief complaint. There may also be drainage of watery fluid or pus into the outer ear canal. Your child's hearing may also be diminished in the affected ear, and he may have fever. However, many children with middle ear infections have few or none of these symptoms.

Infants with middle ear infections may have crying spells, irritability, and decreased appetite. Sometimes infants pull at the ears and wince when the infected ear is touched. Diarrhea may be the only symptom in other infants. Arrange for an early examination by a physician whenever your child shows any of these symptoms. Early treatment usually prevents complications such as hearing loss, mastoiditis, and meningitis. Prolonged or recurrent middle ear infections in infants and preschool children can sometimes cause delay in speech and language development and poor school performance.

Doctors usually prescribe antibiotics for treatment of middle ear infections. If your child is taking antibiotics, it is important for him to stay on the medication for the full amount of time prescribed by your doctor even if his symptoms are quickly alleviated. Antibiotics are usually taken for about 10 days. Arrange for a follow-up visit to make certain that the condition is cured and that you can discontinue the medication.

External Ear Infection

An infection of the external ear canal usually develops in some children who swim or dive for long periods of time in swimming pools or lakes. That's why it is also called "swimmer's ear." Ocean swimming is sometimes involved, but swimming in crowded, warm pools increases the likelihood of this type of ear infection. The infection can affect either a small part of the ear canal lining or the entire canal lining.

Causes. An infection of the external ear canal is usually caused by bacteria that thrive in fresh water. Water that remains in the ear canal provides the right environment for certain bacteria to grow. During prolonged swimming, the water softens and wrinkles the lining of the ear canal; similar to the way your child's fingertips and toes look wrinkled after a long bath. This wrinkling allows the bacteria to penetrate more easily. Dirt or wax in the ear canal can dam up the water and can also promote ear infection. Cotton swabs inserted to clean the ear canal can cause harm by blocking the drainage of water. This is why it's best to clean the outer part of your child's ears only and to use a damp washcloth.

Symptoms. Six hours to five days after swimming, there may be itching, pain, or a "blocked" feeling in the ear. In addition, your child may not be able to hear as well as usual. In severe cases, there may be a foul-smelling, puslike, blood-tinged discharge in the outer ear. The earlobe of the affected area may be very tender to touch, and the pain can become intense with crying and difficulty chewing. The skin of the ear canal may appear red and swollen, and a slight fever may occur. Try to have your child examined by the pediatrician as soon as possible.

What Parents Can Do

- Have the doctor examine your child if he has an earache. Avoid using eardrops before he is examined.
- Have the doctor examine your infant if he becomes very fretful and cries more than usual for several hours or if he has diarrhea for more than one day.
- If your child has an ear infection, make sure to continue giving him antibiotics for the full amount of time prescribed by the doctor. Bring him back to the doctor for a follow-up examination to make sure the infection is completely cleared.
- Although you may be tempted to use cotton swabs or ear drops to clean out your child's ears, avoid doing so. This can aggravate an ear infection.
- If your child spends time swimming and diving in pools, buy him a pair of correct-sized ear plugs. Show him how to properly insert them, and make certain he uses them before swimming.

What the Doctor May Do

- Examine your child's ears to determine whether he has an ear infection.
- Prescribe antibiotics to treat an ear infection.
- Arrange a follow-up visit to reexamine your child's ears and make sure the infection has cleared.
- Arrange for a hearing test after the infection has cleared.

15

~~~~~~

ENURESIS

Occasional urinary incontinence (the inability to retain urine during the day or night) is considered normal in preschool children. It takes a few years after birth for the control center in the brain that controls the bladder muscles to mature fully. Coordination of the nervous system and the bladder represents a balancing act between the storing of urine and the release of it. In some children, increased bladder capacity and nervous system control take a longer time to develop than in other children.

Most children complete their bladder and bowel training by four years of age. But occasional episodes of bedwetting occur in about 30 percent of children up to six years of age. In fact, these occasional wet-bed events are so common in the preschool years that most pediatricians prefer to use the medical term for wetting (enuresis) only when a child is over six years of age.

Frequent bedwetting during sleep is called *nocturnal enuresis*, and it is more common in boys. About 10 percent of six-year-olds have this problem, but by twelve years of age only 3 percent do. Daytime wetting (diurnal enuresis), however, rarely occurs over six years of age; about 1 percent of children, girls as well as boys, experience it.

Types of Enuresis
Enuresis is called *primary* when a child has never had good control of his bladder by the time he reaches six years. Enuresis is called *secondary* when a six-year-old begins regular

bedwetting after he has had a completely dry bed for at least six straight months. About 20 percent of bedwetters have this secondary type, resulting from either physical or psychological causes. Often a history of bedwetting exists in other members of the immediate family.

Causes

There are physical, emotional, and sometimes even situational factors that may cause a child to lose bladder control.

When some children are very absorbed in play or if they withhold their urine too long and can't reach the bathroom on time, they may accidentally wet themselves. A bout of laughter or an emotionally stressful event may also result in wetting in some children. These are situational factors, and the wetting episodes are infrequent.

A physical condition is the cause of enuresis in less than 5 percent of all cases. Physical causes are more likely in secondary enuresis but are still rarely found. A urinary tract infection is the most frequent physical cause. Other less likely physical causes are: diabetes, congenital abnormalities of the lower urinary tract or spine, severe constipation, and urethral irritants such as strong citrus juices or bubble baths. (The urethra is the canal that carries urine from the bladder.)

Psychological problems involving the child, parents, or siblings can also be severe enough to cause enuresis in some young children. Some of these problems are related to feelings of insecurity and a craving for love and attention. Stressful events such as the death of a parent or a divorce may also cause secondary enuresis. Many children experience the birth of a sibling as stressful and feel displaced, less important, or neglected. Psychologists say that regression may occur under stress and that the first thing to go is the last thing that's been learned. It's not unusual, then, for a child who has recently begun to use the toilet to have episodes of wetting (and even soiling) during a difficult emotional time.

It's sometimes frustrating and disappointing to parents when their child starts to wet himself after a period of successful bladder training. However, it's important to muster patience, tolerance, and understanding. Don't assume that your child's behavior is motivated by some malicious intent. He will need even more love and attention during this time.

Signs of Physical Causes

Be alert for any of the following symptoms in your child. They may indicate that his enuresis is caused by a physical problem:

- Painful urination or straining during urination
- Frequent urination during the day
- Dribbling of urine
- Poor bowel control or infrequent bowel movements
- Cloudy or pink urine or blood stains on underpants

Home Management

After six years of age, *primary* enuresis begins to disappear in some children who have it. Generally, physicians don't consider treatment before six years of age unless a physical cause such as a urinary tract infection is found.

Accurate monitoring is the first step in treatment. If your child wets regularly every day or two, keep a written record of the times of the day and the circumstances at those times. For example, note whether he was engaged in a play activity or whether he was being scolded or punished before the wetting accident occurred. Also note in the record whether he had been drinking large amounts of liquids, such as caffeinated soda or tea, before the event and whether he recently ate any spicy food or drank any citrus juices, which sometimes act as irritants.

You may want to use a monitoring chart to help you record all this information. Here's a sample chart:

EPISODES OF WETTING

Day	Time of Day	Circumstance	Intake (What ate, drank, how much, and when)

After a few weeks, show these records to the doctor.

There are several other important things you can do. Check the appearance of the urine regularly to see if there is any pink discoloration or cloudiness. If so, collect a small sample of the urine in a clean jar, refrigerate it, and bring it to the doctor for analysis.

A child with nocturnal enuresis should not be allowed to drink any liquids after dinnertime. Remind your child to use the bathroom right before going to bed. Ask the doctor if he advises waking your child up to urinate in the bathroom about two hours after going to bed. If his bed is dry in the morning, you may praise or reward him but avoid physical or verbal punishment for wetting. Rewarding the positive behavior is more effective and less demoralizing than punishing the negative behavior. Children with enuresis usually feel embarrassed and ashamed about the wetting.

After fully evaluating his history, conducting a physical examination, and taking urine tests, the doctor will decide if, when, and what treatment is advisable. If there is no physical cause for the enuresis, consider consulting a mental health professional (such as a psychologist or psychiatrist) who has expertise in treating this type of problem.

What Parents Can Do

- Don't consider your child a "wetter" unless he wets repeatedly after he is six years old.
- Don't become alarmed if there is occasional wetting. This is normal up to six years of age. Try to pinpoint the circumstances that may have caused the wetting episodes and avoid them in the future.
- If your child becomes a regular "wetter"—especially if it happens day and night—watch for signs of physical causes. Make sure you have a doctor examine him and do a urinalysis.
- Keep written records of the times and conditions of all wetting events if he becomes a regular "wetter" after six years of age. Show these to the doctor at the checkup.
- Use praise for dry beds but avoid punishment for wet ones. The objective is not to create further emotional stress in you and your child, which may only reinforce the condition. Reassurance and patience are best.
- If there is no physical cause for the problem, consider consulting with a mental health professional who has expertise in treating children and families with this problem.

What the Doctor May Do

- Conduct a thorough checkup, including a physical examination, urine analysis, and history taking.
- Review details of your record in order to better understand the episodes of enuresis.
- Recommend beginning steps for home management when indicated.
- Prescribe an antibiotic if a urinary tract infection is determined to be the cause.

16

FOOD POISONING

Children as well as adults can become ill after eating contaminated foods, and the usual symptoms are vomiting, diarrhea, and abdominal pain. This common condition is termed *food poisoning*. Most food poisoning is due to bacteria or viruses, bacterial toxins (chemicals produced by bacteria), or naturally occurring poisons in some foods. When several people have eaten the same contaminated food at the same meal, a food poisoning outbreak may occur.

Some foodborne bacteria grow more rapidly in certain foods, and some toxins are produced only in certain types of food. At times, the contaminated food will taste or smell bad, but often it will not.

Bacterial Causes

Many species of bacteria can contaminate food. *Salmonella* bacteria are among the most common culprits. They can easily grow in milk, eggs, chicken, and meat. If any of these foods are eaten raw or are undercooked or the milk is unpasteurized, there is a high risk of food poisoning. That is why children should never drink raw, unpasteurized milk or eat eggs or chicken dishes that have not been thoroughly cooked or that have been kept out of the refrigerator for more than one hour.

Staphylococcus, another type of bacteria that causes food poisoning, is frequently found in boils and skin infections. If people who handle food have uncovered skin infections on their hands or face, they can easily transmit these bacteria to foods where they can multiply within hours. This is especially true for unrefrigerated foods such as custards, cream-filled pastries, meat, and egg salads. As they grow, the bacteria manufacture a toxin that irritates the cells of the gastrointestinal tract after the food is eaten. Cooking does not destroy this toxin.

Food can also be contaminated by some types of bacterial spores (*B. cereus*). The most common way for this to happen is that the person who prepares the food carries the bacteria in his intestinal tract and does not wash his hands after using the bathroom. The bacterial spores are not killed by normal cooking of meat, poultry, stews, and gravies. They can open and multiply as bacteria during the cooking, storage, or rewarming stages of preparing these foods. These bacteria also produce toxins that resist normal cooking temperatures and cause intestinal illness.

Botulism is also a form of food poisoning. It is caused by another spore-forming species of bacteria and produces a potent toxin in improperly home-canned vegetables and fruits. If these foods are contaminated with the spores and then inadequately cooked (less than several hours of boiling) before canning, toxins form. If these foods are later inadequately heated (less than 15 to 20 minutes of boiling) before eating, the toxin will not be destroyed and will remain in the food when it is eaten. This bacteria can then cause a group of severe gastrointestinal and nervous system symptoms known as botulism.

Honey, whether home-canned or commercial, may contain these spores. If fed to infants, the bacteria germinate from the spores and can cause infantile botulism. Adults can safely eat commercially prepared honey, but infants under one year of age should never be given *any* honey because it can produce fatal botulism.

75

Nonbacterial Causes

Many species of mushrooms growing in the wild contain naturally occurring toxins. Eating these mushrooms can lead to serious symptoms within several minutes to hours. Some plants and shrubs also contain poisonous leaves, flowers, or fruits and pose a danger to children who swallow them. Some examples are morning glory, horse chestnuts, and bird-of-paradise flower.

Toxins can be present in many species of fish, and they cannot be detected by smell or taste. However, many of these toxins are destroyed by adequate cooking. (This is why even though sushi is chic, it's not recommended fare for children.) *Scombroid poisoning* (in fish of the mackerel and tuna families) results from bacterial decomposition in fish that has not been kept cold enough after being caught. A toxin similar to histamine then forms in the fish and causes this serious illness. In addition, intestinal viruses or hepatitis A virus can sometimes be swallowed in shellfish that are not adequately cooked. Steaming is usually not adequate to kill these viruses.

Symptoms

Symptoms usually begin anytime from a few minutes to 48 hours after ingestion of the toxin, depending on the cause of the poisoning. Vomiting, diarrhea, and abdominal pain are the chief symptoms. In addition, salmonella infections can occasionally cause fever and bloody diarrhea, and scombroid poisoning can cause facial flushing and/or hives within a few minutes after eating.

Botulism has symptoms involving the nervous system, in addition to vomiting. Symptoms appear about 12 to 36 hours after ingestion of the toxic food and include:

- Double vision
- Difficulty in swallowing

- Dry mouth
- Breathing difficulty
- Paralysis of various muscles

Infant botulism usually starts with constipation, followed by poor sucking and swallowing, droopy eyelids, weak cry, and generalized "floppiness" (weakness).

Botulism is a life-threatening disease that requires immediate attention in the nearest emergency room. Hospitalization is often necessary for continuous observation and treatment.

Most cases of food poisoning last one to seven days, but complete recovery of the nervous system from botulism may take months.

Prevention

All fruits and vegetables should be thoroughly washed before being eaten. Poultry, meats, seafood, and eggs must be thoroughly cooked to ensure that they are free of harmful bacteria. Don't allow your children to eat raw (unpasteurized) milk, raw meat, or uncooked shellfish (including sushi).

If you are a home-canner, follow the exact time, pressure, and temperature recommended to be certain that the spores that cause botulism are killed. Don't buy and don't open any bulging cans of food. Don't taste and don't eat any foods with "off" odors.

Serve hot meat and poultry dishes soon after they are cooked. If perishable foods must be stored for more than two hours, place them in shallow containers and cover them. They can be stored hot on a stove, grill, or chafing dish or stored cold in the refrigerator. Refrigerate pastries, custards, and salads as soon as possible after they are prepared.

Here are some other important guidelines to prevent food poisoning:

- Wash your hands, the tops of kitchen counters, and cutting boards thoroughly after handling raw meat and raw poultry.
- Don't prepare or handle food if you have any open sores or cuts on your face or hands unless they are completely covered.
- Wear gloves if you have an open infections on your hands.
- Wash your hands with soap and water after using the toilet or changing diapers.
- Don't prepare food for your child if you have diarrhea, vomiting, or abdominal cramps, and don't share food from the same dish as your child if you have these illnesses.

Personal cleanliness and cleanliness in the kitchen are the watchwords.

What Parents Can Do

- Be careful in all your food selection, preparation, and storage.
- Maintain good personal hygiene habits and good sanitation habits in the kitchen.
- Meats, poultry, eggs, and seafood must always be thoroughly cooked and should never be eaten raw or partially raw.
- Never feed honey to your child if she is under one year of age.
- Never give your child unpasteurized milk.
- Don't buy any cans of food that have bulges.
- Don't taste or eat any food with an "off" odor.
- Make sure your child doesn't eat any leaves, flowers, or fruits when she is in the backyard or in the woods.

What the Doctor May Do

- Inquire when the symptoms began and ask for a detailed description of the symptoms.

- Ask whether anyone else in the family has gastrointestinal symptoms (vomiting, diarrhea, abdominal pain) at the same time.
- Ask whether your child recently ate a new dish, had seafood (including shellfish), ate at a restaurant, or was traveling (and where).
- Prescribe medication and recommend a modified diet to alleviate the symptoms.
- Arrange for culture tests of a sample of the child's stool.

17

GERMAN MEASLES (RUBELLA)

I f your child catches German measles (rubella), there isn't reason for alarm. Although it's always upsetting to have an ill child, this is a mild, contagious rash disease that does not have any complications. The only danger is in the case of congenital rubella, in which a pregnant woman has German measles and passes the disease along to the fetus. Congenital rubella is a serious condition because it can lead to death of the fetus or to major defects in the newborn.

Before a rubella vaccine became available in 1969, German measles, or three-day measles, was one of the most common contagious diseases of childhood. Up to that time, epidemics of rubella occurred every six to nine years in the United States. The disease is so contagious that outbreaks in schools or institutions commonly involved almost 100 percent of the children or adults who were not immune.

In the 1990s minor outbreaks of rubella are reported occasionally on college campuses in the United States because up to 20 percent of enrolled students have never had either the vaccine or the disease.

Immunity

Once you have had German measles, you are immune (protected) for life. If you never had the disease but received the rubella vaccine after 12 months of age, you will probably have lifelong immunity, too. However, not every case of rubella is seen and diagnosed by a physician, and many adolescents and young adults mistakenly believe they are immune. That is why it is so critical for all college students and health care workers in hospitals and clinics to have proof of immunity— either a physician-documented history of the disease or an accurate history of rubella immunization. It is also important for women who are planning to get pregnant to know whether they've had the disease.

If you have doubt about whether you have had either the disease or the vaccine, you should have a blood test to see if you have rubella antibodies (immunity). If there are no antibodies, you should receive the vaccine as soon as feasible, unless you are a women in early pregnancy, in which case the vaccine is not advisable.

An infant whose mother is immune to rubella will usually have her antibodies and will be protected for the first six to nine months of life.

Cause
The rubella virus is around all year, but the winter and spring months are the most likely times for it to spread. Your child may catch the virus from droplets in room air coming from the nose or throat secretions of an infected person.

Your child will not show symptoms of the illness until about 14 to 21 days after he has had close contact with an infected person. The disease is most contagious about seven days before and five days after the rash appears, leaving a 12-day span when infection is most likely.

In *congenital rubella*, the virus reaches the fetus through the mother's blood that supplies the womb. The risk of congenital rubella decreases as the pregnancy progresses. During the first three months of pregnancy, if the mother has the disease, there is about a 25 percent chance the fetus will catch it. The risk falls to 10 to 20 percent during the fourth month of pregnancy and to almost zero after the fifth month of pregnancy.

Congenital rubella is a serious disease that can result in birth defects, including damage to the ears, eyes, heart, or neurologic system (brain). As a result, the infant may have permanent deafness, blindness, or mental retardation. Fortunately, there are a dozen or fewer cases of congenital rubella reported in the United States each year.

Symptoms

Children usually begin the illness with a rash, and there is a low-grade fever (101°F) that lasts one day. Older children and adolescents often begin with preliminary symptoms for three or four days. Early symptoms include headache, low fever, sore throat, slight cough, and tender and enlarged lymph glands behind the ears and the head.

The rash begins as pink-red spots on the face. The spots soon spread down to the neck, arms, trunk, and legs. Many cases don't develop any visible rash, which is the reason many adults can be immune without knowing they ever had rubella.

The rash, which doesn't itch, may cover the entire body after the first day. On the second day, it starts to disappear from the face, and it usually fades from the entire body after three days.

The lymph glands behind the ears and head may remain swollen without tenderness for several weeks. Some adolescents may complain of joint (knees, ankles, or elbows) pain as the rash fades. These pains may linger for 10 days.

What Parents Can Do

• Make sure your pediatrician administers the rubella vaccine to your child once she reaches 15 months of age. It is part of the combined measles-mumps-rubella (MMR) vaccine and it is 98 percent effective in producing protective rubella antibody.

- Have your child avoid close contact with any person—child or adult—who has an undiagnosed rash, since it might indicate German measles.
- Don't send your child to a day-care center or school if he has an undiagnosed rash. The doctor must first examine him to decide whether he has a contagious disease such as rubella. If the disease is contagious, ask the doctor how long he recommends that your child be isolated from others.
- If your child comes down with rubella, keep her away from pregnant women for at least 5 days after the rash begins. If there should be accidental contact of this type, the pregnant woman should immediately consult her obstetrician for advice.
- If the doctor diagnoses your child as having rubella, keep her away from all other children for at least five days after the rash began. However, close contact with another child who had previously received the rubella vaccine (MMR) can be allowed since that child has immunity.

What the Doctor May Do

- Establish a correct diagnosis by examining your child and asking questions such as: "When did the rash begin?" "Where did the rash begin?" and "Has your child recently played with a child who had German measles?"
- Immunize your child against rubella by administering the measles-mumps-rubella (MMR) vaccine once your child is over 15 months old.
- If your child has German measles, advise you to keep her at home and isolate her from other children until she is no longer contagious.
- Recommend an over-the-counter medication for the aches and fever.

18

HAY FEVER AND ALLERGIC RHINITIS

Allergic rhinitis (or nasal allergy) is a very troublesome condition for many children. It includes symptoms such as sneezing, runny nose, and itchy nose. If these symptoms occur in spring, summer, or fall, the condition is called *seasonal* allergic rhinitis. (Years ago, it was called *hay fever*.) If the symptoms occur throughout the year, it is known as *perennial* allergic rhinitis.

These illnesses are rare in infants and in children under six years of age. Very young children are more likely to develop food allergies (see Key 5). Hay fever occurs in about 10 percent of all school-aged children and results in many school absences each year. Many of these children have a parent with a history of allergic rhinitis or asthma, which suggests that this condition is often inherited.

The substances or allergens to which some children are sensitive (such as dust or tree pollens) may be present in the outdoor environment in some geographic locations. They may also be present in the home, in the form of dust, feathers, or dog dander (tiny skin sheddings).

Fortunately, most children with nasal allergies show clear improvement by the time they reach late adolescence or young adulthood. My older son, for example, suffered terribly with nasal allergies, but his condition was greatly alleviated as he matured.

Causes

When an allergen in the environment repeatedly contacts the mucous membrane (inner lining) of the nose, some allergy-prone children gradually produce a specific antibody to it. This specific allergen and its specific antibody later bind to certain cells in the nasal membrane and cause the release of a chemical called histamine. Histamine causes swelling of the lining of the membranes in the nose and increases the mucus secretion of its cells.

In the spring (May and June) in the United States, allergic rhinitis can occur in children sensitive to the pollens of various trees such as oaks, elms, or maples. In the summer (June and July), grass pollens such as Bermuda or meadow grass or weed pollens like English plantain can be the causative allergens. From mid-August to mid-September, ragweed pollen counts are high and can trigger hay fever in some children and adolescents.

Surprisingly, the indoor environment of the average household contains many potential allergens. Ordinary house dust is the most common one that is present all year round. You can find dust in each and every home regardless of how clean it is kept. Some dust is always present in mattresses, rugs and carpets, blankets, upholstery, stuffed animals, and unfiltered air from the furnace. Feathers are another common allergen that can be found in pillows, blankets, and upholstered furniture. Molds (microscopic fungi) grow indoors in damp cellars, attics, closets, and mattresses. They also grow outdoors in dark, damp areas in the lawn or garden.

Some children are also allergic to certain pets such as dogs, cats, or birds. Tropical fish usually are no problem. Certain breeds of dogs or certain dogs within a given breed can cause more allergic sensitivities than others. It doesn't matter whether the dog is long-haired or short-haired, because the nasal allergy is caused not by their shed hair but rather by the dander.

Symptoms

If your child is suffering from allergic rhinitis, you may think he has a common cold. At the onset, these conditions look alike. But when your child has a cold or upper respiratory infection, the clear watery secretions of the nose become thick and yellow or green after a couple of days. With seasonal allergic rhinitis, the nasal secretions remain clear and any of the following symptoms can develop and continue for days, weeks, or months:

• Sneezing
• Watery, runny nose or stuffy nose
• Itching of eyes, nose, or throat
• Coughing
• Tearing, swollen, or red eyes
• Headaches

In addition to these symptoms, "allergic shiners" (dark circles under the eyes), "allergic salute" (rubbing the nose), mouth breathing, or night snoring can occur.

The symptoms of perennial allergic rhinitis can vary from month to month and from day to day. In these cases, the children complain mostly of stuffy nose and often breathe with an open mouth. Perennial allergies rhinitis can lead to sinusitis, middle ear infections, or hearing problems.

Chronic nasal allergies often interfere with sleep and appetite, and your child can become very cranky. I clearly remember my own son at the age of 10 experiencing a very rough summer with his nasal allergy. In despair, he begged me one day: "Dad, cut off my nose!" But he kept his troublesome nose, and it improved slowly during his adolescence.

86

What Parents Can Do

- If possible, purchase an air conditioner or air filter for your child's room. Most children with nasal allergies feel better when they breathe air under these conditions.
- If your child has a continuous runny nose with sneezing or stuffiness for more than one week, take him to the doctor. Don't buy antiallergy medications or nose sprays because they may make the symptoms worse.
- To relieve your child's discomfort, administer the antihistamines the doctor prescribes.
- With a child who is old enough to understand, teach him about his allergies and reassure him that his symptoms will improve.

What the Doctor May Do

- If the doctor diagnoses allergic rhinitis, he will prescribe an antihistamine and possibly other medications to relieve your child's symptoms.
- If the medications the doctor prescribes are not effective enough, he may change them or he may refer your child to an allergist for skin or blood testing.
- The allergist will try to pinpoint the allergen(s) causing your child's symptoms. If it is dust, feathers, or molds, he will instruct you on how best to eliminate them in the home. He may also advise other forms of treatment such as desensitization injections. If you closely follow his advice, it is likely that you will see a dramatic improvement in your child's symptoms.

19

HEAD LICE

I f you ever notice white specks stuck to your child's hairs and these specks can't be removed like dandruff, he may have head lice. Although the idea can be upsetting, try not to become too excited because this condition is easily treated.

Before you call the doctor, call the school nurse or day-care director to find out if there have been any cases of head lice reported recently in any children.

Many parents become irate if they learn that several cases have occurred in their child's class. Some of them call the principal and demand that a full-scale hair examination be done on every child in the school every day. Others demand an emergency PTA meeting. (Sometimes this condition can result in unjustified parental hysteria.)

I am familiar with this reaction not only as a pediatrician but as a parent. Once, when there was an outbreak of head lice in my children's elementary school, my daughter's teacher panicked and urged us to cut off her long hair. The outbreak soon subsided, and her long hair remained uncut.

It is probable that every school in the United States at one time or another has experienced cases of head lice. In the first quarter of this century, head lice were common in children, and many schools conducted daily head inspections in every classrooms. Today, large outbreaks in school are rare, but clusters of cases occur occasionally in some schools and day-care centers. More often, a few isolated cases appear in both high- and low-income communities and both suburban and city schools.

Causes

The six-legged, diamond-shaped louse found on the head is technically called *Pediculus capitis*. Grayish-white and about two millimeters long, it can travel from person to person directly through head-to-head contact or indirectly by the sharing of hats, hair ribbons, combs, or brushes. The nits (eggs) of the female louse can survive on clothing and upholstered chairs (such as those in theaters and auditoriums) for seven days. But the lice can live for only two days away from a head, and they're communicable only while they're alive.

Symptoms

Children who have few lice (one to five) may have slight itching of the scalp, while others may not complain at all. If you look closely, you may see the tiny white nits attached to the hair close to the scalp, especially near the back of the neck. The nits may resemble dandruff flakes stuck to the hair shaft. On rare occasions, if there is heavy infestation, you may see a slow-crawling louse. Bring your child to the doctor for the diagnosis (he may need a magnifying glass or microscope, if in doubt) and for medicated shampoo treatment.

You can tell how long the nits have been present on the hairs. Nits that are one centimeter or more from the scalp have probably been on the hair for at least two weeks. After treatment, the nits will be dead and you can remove them with a fine-toothed comb.

Prevention & Control

Keep your child out of school or day care if she has nits or lice. You can send her back the day after she has the special shampoo treatment with a note from the doctor saying she was treated. Any remaining nits that may be seen are no longer alive or communicable.

It's necessary for the school or day-care center to become aware of your child's lice problem. The school nurse or day-care staff will then examine all close contacts of your child for head lice or nits. They can then refer any child who has them to the doctor.

Several different medicated shampoos are available to treat lice and nits. After the doctor recommends one for your child, follow the directions carefully. A single shampoo will treat the hair for two weeks, but some doctors repeat the shampoo after seven days.

Machine-wash (hot) and -dry all hats and scarves recently worn by your child if she is diagnosed with lice. Do the same with her sheets and pillowcases. This will prevent recurrence. Combs and hairbrushes should be washed with the same shampoo solution you used for her head.

What Parents Can Do

- If your child has an itchy scalp, carefully look for nits or lice. If you think you see any or are in doubt, take her to the doctor.
- If your child has lice, don't panic, and try not to feel guilty or ashamed. Lice can be found in any family anywhere— even if they maintain good personal hygiene. Lice can be easily caught from others, and their presence doesn't necessarily mean poor hygiene in your child.
- Head lice are easy to treat. The day after you give your child the specially medicated shampoo and fine-tooth combing, you can send her back to her school or day-care center with a doctor's note.
- Machine-wash your child's hats in hot water and thoroughly wash her comb, brush, hair clips, and headbands.
- Contact the school nurse and ask her if there is an outbreak of head lice in the school.

What the Doctor May Do

- Examine your child's hair and scalp. Use a magnifying glass or microscope, if in doubt.
- Prescribe a medicated shampoo.
- Provide a note for the school or day-care center indicating that your child has had treatment and is ready to return.
- Examine all other members of the family for nits or lice and prescribe treatment for them, if necessary. This would include hot-water washing of their bedding, hats, combs, and hair brushes.
- Advise repeating the medicated shampoo about one week later.

20

~~~~~~

HERPES SIMPLEX INFECTIONS

B etween the ages of one and four years, your child may develop a viral infection in his mouth caused by the *herpes simplex virus* (HSV). If this happens, he will have tiny, clear blisters or open sores. The infection caused by this virus is a communicable disease that is especially common in children of low-income families who live under crowded conditions. More than half the population becomes infected with this virus during childhood or young adulthood. All these people then become lifelong carriers of the virus and its antibody. However, they are contagious only when the virus is in the active stage.

There are two different types of herpes simplex virus that affect different parts of the body. The virus you are most likely to encounter is the one that causes blisters in your child's mouth. Although this can be painful and can recur, it is not a serious illness.

Cause

The two major types of herpes simplex virus that generally cause infections are HSV-1 and HSV-2. The virus that usually infects the body above the waist is HSV-1. The virus that usually is manifest below the waist (on the skin or the genitalia) and that can infect a newborn during birth is HSV-2.

After the infection clears, the virus continues to survive in a latent (dormant) state in the local nerve cells of the mucous membranes or the skin. A person who is infected may become a lifetime carrier of the virus. (About 50 percent of adults carry the virus, but they're not contagious, unless the herpes is active.) Months or years later, the HSV lesions may recur whenever there is a triggering event such as strong sunlight exposure, fever, injury, or psychological stress. They are sometimes called "cold sores" or "fever blisters."

More than half of all newborns have their mother's HSV antibodies and are immune to the disease until they're about six months old. Unlike many other viral diseases of childhood, an HSV infection doesn't guarantee lifetime immunity against future HSV infections. This means that your child can get HSV more than once. However, it's hard to tell whether an infection is new (primary) or reactivated (recurrent).

The HSV-1 virus is present in the saliva, skin, lesions, urine, and stools of the infected child or adult. Saliva spread by kissing or by sharing eating utensils or food is the most common transmitter of HSV-1.

The HSV-2 virus is acquired through sexual contact and affects the genital area.

Symptoms

In many children, the primary infection with HSV-1 does not produce any symptoms. In others, especially those between one and four years of age, it may begin as an acute inflammation of the gums and mouth (acute gingivo-stomatitis). It can also begin quickly with a fever (low or high), sore mouth, and loss of appetite. Clear blisters called vesicles appear on the lips, gums, tongue, palate, or mucous membranes lining the mouth. Many of these vesicles soon break and look like small, white plaques or ulcers. The gums swell and look red, and salivation increases. At times, the vesicles may spread to the skin around the nose or mouth and back into the throat or into the area around the tonsils. Often there's pain and difficulty in chewing and swallowing. If you notice this happening with your child, ask the pediatrician for medication to apply to the *lesions*—or blisters—to help relieve your child's irritability or discomfort.

The illness lasts one week or longer with or without fever, but the virus (HSV) can remain in the saliva and be contagious for several weeks. This means that even though your child may no longer have symptoms or experience discomfort, he can still pass the infection on to others during this time period.

Eye lesions due to HSV-1 are rare and can appear at any age. These usually affect the cornea (the tissue on the front part of the eyeball), conjunctiva (lining of the eyelids and eyeball), or eyelid on one side only. Fever and a pus-like discharge appear along the vesicles on the eyelid. The condition usually clears in about two weeks, but antiviral medication is necessary to prevent permanent damage to vision.

Children who have allergic eczema on rare occasions may acquire herpes virus infections in their eczema skin lesions. If your child has this type of allergic skin disorder, she should avoid physical contact with people who have HSV infections.

Infections caused by HSV-2 can be serious. The rare newborn who becomes infected with HSV-2 is usually of low birthweight. If the mother of an infant born by vaginal delivery is experiencing an HSV genital infection (a first infection), the chances are about 50 percent that the infant will develop *neonatal* (or newborn) HSV infection.

There are three major forms of neonatal—or newborn—HSV-2 infection that can appear during the first few weeks after birth:

- Generalized infection involving internal organs such as the liver or lungs or brain (encephalitis)
- Infection of the brain (encephalitis) only with fever and convulsions
- Infection of the skin, eyes, or mouth

All of these forms of neonatal HSV infection require immediate hospitalization and antiviral medication to prevent permanent damage or death.

Genital herpes can develop in adolescents (male and female) with HSV-2 but is rare in children. These infections have painful ulcers along with fever and can last up to 20 days. More than half of these cases later have milder recurrences, each lasting a few days.

Whether a person has HSV-1 or HSV-2, there are secondary (recurrent) infections that occur all through childhood and adolescence. Lesions can appear on the lips or around the mouth at the same locations as the primary (original) lesions that appeared months or years before. Except for mild pain, they usually cause few symptoms.

What Parents Can Do

- Protect your child from HSV infections by doing the following:
  - Don't allow anyone with sores, scabs, or blisters around the mouth or nose to kiss your child.
  - Make sure infected people don't share food or eating utensils with her.
- If your child develops any tiny blisters around the eyes or eyelids, bring her to the doctor for a diagnosis.
- If your child has a herpes infection, speak to the doctor about lotions, ointments, or medication you can use to relieve discomfort.

- If your child has an HSV infection, keep her out of school or day care until her skin, mouth, lip, and eye have completely healed. This may take at least one or two weeks.
- If your child has a history of recurrent HSV, protect her around the nose or mouth with sun-blocking lotions before she has long exposure to summer sunlight.

What the Doctor May Do

- If your child has the HSV infection, your pediatrician may prescribe medication to apply to the lesions or medication to help relieve her irritability or discomfort.
- The doctor will hospitalize a newborn infant (birth to 30 days) with HSV infection and treat her quickly with antiviral medication.
- In the case of a woman of childbearing age who has genital HSV infection, the doctor may prescribe antiviral medication.
- In the case of a pregnant woman with genital HSV late in pregnancy, her doctor may recommend delivery by cesarean section.

21

~~~~~~

LEAD POISONING

If you have a young child, you may have heard the doctor mention the need to administer a *blood lead screening test* and wondered what this was about. Although the need for this type of screening has only recently been recognized, lead has been known to be a poisonous chemical all the way back to ancient Roman times. If swallowed or inhaled, lead can cause serious damage to the brain, nervous system, and kidneys. Although lead poisoning can occur at any age, it is most common in children from six months to six years of age. Those under two years old are at the highest risk.

In the last 20 years or so, many thousands of children in the United States have been found to have dangerous levels of lead in their blood (a disease medically referred to as *plumbism*). Most of these children live in poor urban areas, but others do not. For example, a national study recently showed that 55 percent of poor and African-American children and 12 percent of rich or middle-class children suffer from the mental effects of excess lead. Even if you fall in the latter group, this is still an important disease for you to know about.

Regardless of income, parents who live in old houses should be aware of the potential risks of plumbism from old paint or old pipes.

Children get lead poisoning by:

- Ingesting lead-based paint or plaster chips
- Inhaling lead-containing dust, soil, or air
- Drinking lead-contaminated water.

As a parent, you play a key role in checking your old house for peeling paint, cracked ceilings, and lead in the drinking water. Prevention and *early detection* are essential in averting lead poisoning in your children.

Effects of Lead on Brain

If your child regularly swallows or inhales small amounts of lead (other than the tiny amount normally found in some foods), the lead gradually accumulates in his body because it's poorly excreted. The body is not able to process or to get rid of this toxic substance.

The brain and the nervous system are very sensitive to lead. Plumbism can cause serious damage when it occurs in infants and in children under six years old. When pregnant women have high levels of lead in their blood, the fetus is affected. Fetuses and young children are most at risk because the brain structures develop most rapidly before birth and up to six years of age. When a child has lead poisoning that has not been treated, you may see any of these symptoms by the time she reaches preschool or kindergarten:

• Short attention span
• Behavioral problems
• Reading and learning disabilities
• Slow reaction time.

Most cases of lead poisoning are mild, and the effects are reversible once the condition is detected and treated. However, if a child has severe lead poisoning that is not treated promptly, her intelligence and learning abilities will be compromised. Permanent mental and physical retardation can result.

You and your doctor may not suspect slight plumbism at its early stage because most children don't have any acute symptoms like a bellyache or vomiting. That's why the blood lead screening test is so important. The test is first given when a child is six to 12 months old and is periodically repeated until she is six years old. All children who live in or frequently visit houses built before 1960 should have lead screening tests. Even if you do not live in an old apartment or house, it's a good idea to inquire about the building where your child attends play group, day care, or school so that you know whether she should be tested.

If your doctor finds high levels of lead in your child's blood, he may recommend a few days of chemical treatment (called *chelation therapy*) in the hospital to remove much of the accumulated lead from her body. Chelation therapy is not a painful procedure, and keep in mind that only a small percentage of children—those with high blood lead levels—require it. This treatment applies to fewer than 10 percent of these children.

Sources of Lead

Most cases of lead poisoning occur in young children who live in houses built before 1960 that are poorly maintained. Some of these have a craving (*pica*) to eat old lead-based paint or plaster chips that fall from the walls, window sills, radiators, or ceilings. Others may swallow or inhale lead-containing dust, soil, or air inside or outside their house.

Since 1977, the federal government has had strict regulations on the amount of lead permitted in indoor paint. This has been of great help in reducing the amounts of lead present in the air, dust, and soil around the average home. However, not all cases of lead poisoning occur in old, deteriorating houses and apartments. Another common way of getting lead poisoning is by drinking contaminated water in the home. In fact, recent studies have shown that up to 20 percent of young children who have too much lead in the blood have gotten it from drinking lead-containing water in their own homes.

How does this happen? The usual way that lead contaminates the water in the home is by *soft, acidic water* corroding the lead pipes or lead solder that some buildings contain. Lead in the drinking water can be a problem in houses built before 1930 or in fairly new houses built before 1987. Here's why: Before 1930, most plumbing pipes contained lead. Although copper pipes were used in most buildings after that time, plumbers still used lead solder. That's why pipe corrosion continues to cause lead to enter drinking water in many areas of the country that have soft water. As of 1987, the use of lead solder has been illegal in the United States.

Signs of Lead in Water

It's important for you to keep in mind that you can't see, taste, or smell lead. In order to determine whether the water in your house is contaminated, you need to have it tested through a private, qualified laboratory or through your local health department.

As parents, you should suspect lead in your water if:

- Plumbing pipes are dull gray and scratch easily with a house key.
- You see signs of corrosion, such as rust-colored water or staining of dishes or laundry.

Even if you don't see these signs but you live in an old house, you may want to have the water tested. You don't have anything to lose, and it will set you at ease. Your local health department has a list of approved water-testing laboratories.

What Parents Can Do

In order to protect your child's health, it's important for you to be on the lookout for sources of lead in your home and to take the following preventive measures:

- If you suspect the water in your home may be contaminated with lead, arrange for an approved water-testing laboratory to check it out.
- If laboratory tests show a high level of lead in your water, take the following precautions: Avoid drinking or cooking with water that's been in your plumbing system for more than six hours (overnight or during an entire work day). Before using water, let the cold water run for about three minutes. Do this at all faucets that are used for cooking or drinking water.
- If laboratory tests show a high level of lead in your water, never cook with or drink water from the hot-water tap, because hot water dissolves lead from the pipes more quickly than cold water does. Don't use the hot-water tap for preparing baby formulas.
- If you have any plumbing repairs or additions done in the house, make sure the plumber uses only leadfree pipes and solder.
- If you live in an old, high-rise apartment building, flushing the cold water faucets may not remove all the lead. You should buy bottled water if tests show a high lead level.
- In houses built before 1960, repair all cracks and peelings in walls, ceilings, window sills, and radiators. As soon as possible, structures should be professionally scraped and repaired and then repainted or wallpapered. If you rent your home, the landlord may be legally responsible for necessary repairs. Check with your local health department.
- If your infant or young child has been living in a house built before 1960, have her blood level screened by the doctor. Begin lead screening tests at six to 12 months of age.
- If you have a young child, wash her hands regularly before each meal to remove any lead-containing dust, dirt, or old paint that she may have picked up during play in the house or outside.

- If you have an infant, wash her toys and pacifiers regularly.
- Wet-mop hard-surface floors, window sills, and baseboards at least once a week with a high-phosphate detergent solution (such as automatic dishwashing detergent). Don't vacuum these hard surfaces because that will disperse dust that may contain lead.

What the Doctor May Do

- If you live in a house built before 1960 or frequently visit such a house, the doctor may administer the first blood lead screening test sometime between six and 12 months of age. He will continue to administer such tests on a regular basis until your child is six years old.
- The blood lead screening test may be repeated every three to four months if the first tests showed a lead level higher than normal.
- If the blood lead level is at a certain point, the doctor may advise a short hospitalization for medical evaluation of possible lead poisoning. Once it is confirmed that your child has lead poisoning, the doctor may advise a few days of special treatment (chelation therapy) in the hospital.
- If the blood lead level is above normal, the doctor may notify the local health department to inspect and test the house or apartment to determine the exact sources of lead. The sources must then be removed by you and your landlord as soon as possible—according to local public health laws and regulations.

22

^^^

LYME DISEASE
AND TICKS

Lyme disease is a serious illness that can result in chronic arthritis and neurologic symptoms if it's not diagnosed and treated early. Physicians in Old Lyme, Connecticut, described the first cases in 1975. However, during the last decade almost all states of the United States have reported cases of this disease, which occurs in both children and adults.

To protect you and your children, it is essential that you know all about the tick that causes Lyme disease and that you be aware of tick-infested areas during the warm seasons, especially in the summer months. Preventive measures work well and should be used regularly for children of all ages who walk or play in those areas.

About the Disease

Corkscrew-shaped bacteria (*Borrelia*) cause the disease, and a tiny tick called *Ixodes* (pronounced ix-ó-deez) carries and spreads it to humans and animals. Any time between three and 32 days after the tick bites, a skin rash appears. The tick bite appears as a small, circular, red patch or pimple on the part of the body where the bite occurred. The skin lesion is technically called *erythema migrans*, or EM. It gradually increases in size to anywhere from two to 20 inches in diameter. As it enlarges, the center of it clears to look like a bull's-eye.

103

Along with the EM lesion, there are other signs to look for, such as fatigue, headache, mild stiff neck, and muscle and joint pains that may last for weeks if antibiotic treatment is not given. Lyme disease is very serious, because within weeks to months after the EM, abnormalities may develop involving the brain or the nerves. About six months after the EM, joint swelling and pain (arthritis) may occur in large joints such as the knee. In a small percentage of cases, heart abnormalities may also develop within a few weeks after the EM.

It's important for you to bring your child to the pediatrician right away if you suspect he has Lyme disease. If the disease is not treated with an antibiotic during the early stages, the arthritis and the neurologic symptoms may recur for years. Blood antibody tests are often necessary to help make the diagnosis but are not always reliable in the early phases of the disease, because the antibodies are not detectable until three or four weeks after the infection begins.

Deer, field mice, and other wild animals that live in wooded areas may carry these ticks on their skin. The ticks then hop onto your child as he walks in the tall grass where these animals have been. However, the Lyme disease bacteria usually spread to humans and animals only after the tick has been attached to the skin for 24 hours or longer. This is why it's critical for you to examine your child's skin right after he has been out in the yard or taken a walk in the woods.

About the Tick

Ixodes is an oval-shaped, eight-legged, dark red and black bug about the size of a pinhead. Unable to fly or jump, it hides in low vegetation of grasslands or wooded areas. It does not cause any pain, swelling, or itching after it silently attaches to the skin of passing animals or humans. If it bites, it gradually swells with the blood of the host and appears much larger. After several hours or days of being attached to the skin, the tick may fall off without the victim ever having noticed it.

There are other ticks in the outdoors that don't cause Lyme disease. For example, there are dog ticks and wood ticks, and they may all look alike to the untrained eye.

Preventive Measures

Like a good scout, prepare for ticks whenever you walk in parks and woods between May and August. Here is what you can do to protect yourself and your family:

- Spray an insect repellent that contains permethrin or DEET (read label on containers) on your child's pants, socks, shoes, and shirt sleeves according to the label directions. Also apply a small amount of the repellent containing DEET (no more than 30 percent) to the back of the neck and to exposed parts of your child's arms and legs every one to two hours. Do not apply it to your child's face or hands or to irritated or scraped skin. Wash DEET off your child's skin after he comes indoors.
- Dress your child in a long-sleeved shirt, tape the cuffs around his wrists, and tuck the shirt into long pants. Tuck the cuffs of the pants into the socks, shoes, or hiking boots. (Your child should not wear open-topped boots.) Dress him in light-colored clothing that has a woven or hard-pressed finish so that you can spot the ticks more easily and so they will not stick to the clothes.
- Watch for warning signs along nature trails and in parks indicating the presence of ticks in the area. Walk near the center of well-cleared paths, trails, and roads whenever possible. Carry a large, white bath towel when hiking in the woods, and drag it along the path frequently during the hike. It ticks are plentiful in the area, you will see many of them as black specks on the white towel.

- Do a body search for ticks on everyone (including the dog) who walked with you as soon as you leave the woodlands. Do a more complete body inspection that night after showering, and wash the removed clothing.

It is especially important to examine your child's ankles, hands, back of the head and scalp, and other parts of his body that may have been in contact with shrubs and underbrush. I remember once finding a tick "hidden" on the back of my daughter's ear after she had been playing in our yard.

When you repeat the body search in your home at night, use a good light.

Tick Removal

If you find a tick on your child's skin, remove it quickly using special precautions. Try not to crush it or kill it because it needs to be properly identified as an Ixodes tick or a non-Lyme-disease-carrying tick.

Don't remove the tick with your bare fingers. Use clean, fine-tipped tweezers (such as those used for eyebrows) to grasp it firmly around its front (mouth) part, and steadily pull it off. If you do not have tweezers, use a facial tissue or a plastic glove for the removal.

Use a magnifying glass to examine the spot where the tick was attached. See if there is any part of the tick that remains embedded. If so, also remove that part with the tweezers. Clean the area of the skin where the tick was attached with an antiseptic solution or with soap and water. Wash your fingers if they were in contact with the tick.

Then place the removed tick—whether dead or alive—into a small, closed container or jar. Call you doctor or your local health department to find out where to bring the tick for identification. If it proves to be a tick other than the

Lyme-disease type, it cannot be a carrier of the Lyme disease bacteria. If it is the dog-tick type, it may be the carrier of a different disease or it may be harmless. Then call the doctor for further advice.

What Parents Can Do

- Learn all you can about the tick that causes Lyme disease and practice good preventive measures as outlined in this chapter. Follow these precautions not only for your child but also for yourself. Parents are important, too!
- Ask your pediatrician to show you a picture of the tick that carries Lyme disease so that you are able to identify it.
- When your child is old enough to understand, teach him about Lyme disease and how to dress when walking in a grassy or wooded area.
- If you find a tick on your child, follow the tick removal procedures as described in this Key and contact your pediatrician.
- If you find a small circular red patch or pimple on your child's body or if he shows any signs such as fatigue, headache, fever, mild stiff neck, or muscle or joint pain, call your pediatrician.

What the Doctor May Do

- Remove the tick (if present) and have it sent to a lab to be identified.
- Take a blood antibody test to help make a diagnosis.
- Prescribe antibiotics to treat Lyme disease and medication to help alleviate any aches and pains. The antibiotics are usually prescribed for 10 to 20 days.

23

MEASLES

Measles (rubeola) is one of the most contagious and serious rash diseases of childhood. Before a measles vaccine became licensed in 1963, almost half a million cases occurred in the United States each year. About every two years there was a major epidemic (outbreak) of the disease, and many deaths followed complicated cases. By the time children became young adults, over 90 percent of them had experienced measles. It seemed as if almost everyone caught it at some point unless she lived on a deserted island or an isolated farm.

Widespread measles immunization programs in the United States since 1963 have reduced the number of measles cases by 98 percent. Each year, however, the disease occurs in some infants under 15 months of age and in many never-immunized preschool children living in inner cities. Occasional outbreaks still happen on some college campuses because some students were never completely immunized against measles as young children. Some of these outbreaks can be traced to foreign students who emigrate to the United States from countries where measles immunization programs are uncommon.

Almost all infants receive measles antibody from their mothers that protects them for about six months after birth. Low levels of this antibody may remain for another six to nine months and can interfere with the effectiveness of an injected measles virus vaccine. For that reason, the measles vaccine is not recommended until infants reach 15 months of age.

After having the disease or after receiving adequate doses of the vaccine, children become protected for life.

Cause

Measles is caused by the rubeola virus that lives in the blood, nose, and throat of people who become infected with it. It spreads easily to other people by way of nose and throat secretions. Coughs and sneezes spray the virus several feet into the surrounding air in the form of microscopic water droplets. These droplets float in the air and are soon inhaled by other people nearby, especially indoors.

As is true for many communicable diseases, most cases of measles occur in winter and early spring for three possible reasons. First, during cold seasons, windows are usually kept closed, and little fresh air enters homes to replace the stale room air that may contain viruses. Second, people who are sick carry viruses indoors during the cold months, which results in their being close to uninfected people. Third, the measles virus (like many others) has difficulty surviving the high temperatures of late spring, summer, and early fall.

Measles is contagious from two days before to five days after the rash appears.

Symptoms

About 10 days after a child is exposed to measles (incubation period), these coldlike symptoms appear:

- Cough
- Runny nose
- Bloodshot eyes and swollen eyelids
- Fever rising from 100° to 103° F

About four days later, a red rash (spots and blotches) begins on the face. The child looks and feels terrible, and his temperature rises to 103° to 105° F for a couple of days as the rash spreads downward to his neck, arms, trunk, and finally his legs. By the fourth day, the rash will remain on his legs and feet while his upper body will have cleared. The rash will completely disappear by the fifth day. Temperature usually returns to normal about two to three days after the rash began, and the harsh cough lingers for several more days.

All children with measles should be under the watchful care of their doctor because several complications can occur. The most frequent are:

• Middle ear infections
• Pneumonia
• Croup

If given early enough, antibiotics are usually effective in treating these complications. Any child with croup should be seen quickly by the doctor. (See Key 12 for more on croup.

Encephalitis (inflammation of the brain) is a rare complication of measles that can develop after the rash appears. It occurs in about one in every 1,000 (0.1 percent) children with measles. Unfortunately, it can result in brain damage or death in those children who contract it.

Measles is a very tiring disease for the sick child and his parents. The child may not be up to returning to school or the day-care center five days after the rash began even though he is no longer contagious at that point.

This dangerous disease is totally preventable by making sure your child is vaccinated early in childhood.

What Parents Can Do

• Call the doctor to examine your child whenever he develops any rash with a fever. The correct diagnosis of all rash diseases during childhood is necessary for ensuring the proper care of the disease and for future reference. Therefore, you should keep a written record of childhood diseases, along with the dates and the name of the doctor(s) who diagnosed them. (See Appendix B.)

- Keep your child out of school or day care for at least five days after the measles rash begins. Make sure that any other children who were close to him had the vaccine when younger or that they go to their doctor for a protective injection.

- Have your healthy child immunized at 15 months of age with the first dose of the measles virus vaccine.

- Get your child a booster (second dose) of the measles virus vaccine when he's five years old (entering kindergarten) or when he's 11 or 12 years old (entering middle or junior high school).

- If your child has not yet been immunized and comes close to a child with measles, call the doctor immediately. Depending on the number of days passed since his exposure to the sick child, the doctor will decide whether to give him the vaccine or an injection of gamma globulin.

- If you have an infant six to 15 months old who becomes exposed to a person with measles or if you live in a community where a measles outbreak is occurring, bring him quickly to the doctor for an injection.

- If your child received his first and only dose of the measles virus vaccine before his first birthday, get him another dose of the vaccine soon after he reaches 15 months of age. He will also need a booster dose before entering kindergarten or middle school.

What the Doctor May Do

- Advise bed rest for your child if he is running a fever.
- Recommend a soft or liquid diet until your child no longer has a fever.

111

- Recommend using acetaminophen for fever or headache.
- Recommend a cough medicine or decongestant.
- Advise you to cleanse any secretions around your child's eyelids with warm water or eye drops.
- Advise bed rest during the few days of moderate to high fever.
- Recommend a soft or liquid diet during the first few days of the rash and fever.
- Prescribe an antibiotic if a secondary bacterial infection of the middle ear or lungs develops.
- Advise you to keep your child indoors, at home, for at least five days after the onset of the rash. After that point, he may associate with other children.

24

MENINGITIS

Meningitis is an inflammation or an infection of the tissues covering the brain and the spinal cord. This is a serious disease, with symptoms such as a high fever, headache, and stiff neck.

It's important to keep in mind that there are two main types of meningitis: *bacterial* and *viral*. These are completely different illnesses with respect to seriousness and outcome. Bacterial meningitis is usually more serious than viral meningitis, and complications involving the brain and the nervous system occur more often following the bacterial type.

Fortunately, neither type of meningitis occurs often. Most of the time, this disease strikes children under five years old, although it can affect children or adults of any age. Children under two years old are especially susceptible to meningitis and usually have the most severe cases with complications.

If diagnosed and treated early in the hospital, about 90 percent of children with meningitis survive, and relatively few survivors have permanent damage to their nervous system. Hearing loss is the most common resulting damage.

Occasional epidemics occur. Most of the time, bacterial meningitis appears in the cool months of the year, while viral meningitis is more common in late summer and early fall.

Causes

Many different types of bacteria can cause this infectious disease, but most cases of bacterial meningitis in childhood are due to these bacteria: *meningococcus, H. influenzae type b*, or *pneumococcus*. A variety of different viruses—especially the *enteroviruses*—can also cause meningitis. Cases of viral meningitis are usually mild, and infected children recover completely in a short time.

The bacterial type of meningitis spreads through contact with people who have the illness or who are carriers (in their nose or throat) of the bacteria. When people who are infected cough or sneeze, microscopic droplets of the bacteria get sprayed in the air and can float there for hours (especially in indoor air). A child who is nearby has the greatest risk for catching the infections after he inhales these droplets. The bacteria then begins to grow in his nose and throat and later spread into the bloodstream. From the blood, the bacteria reach the brain and spinal cord, where they set up the infection.

Most infants are protected against these bacteria for about three months by the antibodies they receive from their mother at birth. Up to 25 percent of the general population of children and adults at times can carry the meningococcus bacteria in their noses or throats for weeks or months without having any symptoms. A similar percentage of the general population can carry the *H. influenzae* bacteria without being ill. Healthy carriers, who far outnumber the actual cases of meningitis, develop lifelong antibodies against these bacteria. It is these carriers, however, who can spread the infections to susceptible people close to them.

Children or adults who come down with mild upper respiratory infections (URI) caused by these bacteria can spread them to others. A few of these contacts may develop meningitis, but most of them will come down with URIs. In either case, all will develop lifelong antibody protection against these dangerous bacteria.

Occasionally bacterial meningitis can result from an infected head injury, sinus infection, or middle ear infection.

Bacterial meningitis is contagious from the onset of symptoms until 24 hours after the start of the high-dose antibiotic treatment.

Viral meningitis is also spread by people with meningitis or by carriers of the virus. It is less contagious than bacterial meningitis. Usually the virus is a common type that infects the gastrointestinal tract. It enters by the mouth and may not completely leave the intestinal tract for several weeks after the child has fully recovered from the meningitis. No antibiotic treatment is effective in killing these viruses, which can spread from the intestinal tract to the brain by way of the bloodstream. Fortunately, they usually do not cause any brain damage.

Symptoms of Bacterial Meningitis

After an incubation period of two to four days, URI symptoms (cough or runny nose) may start. But sometimes the onset is very sudden and progresses rapidly to a stupor or coma within a few hours.

A child will complain of severe headache, along with nausea, vomiting, fever, and chills. His neck may be stiff, and he may also become very irritable, restless, or drowsy. The vomiting is often projectile, which means the vomit shoots out of the mouth with force. The drowsiness may deepen, and the fever may rise rapidly. If you see this happening to your child, bring him to the doctor or the emergency room of the hospital immediately.

Symptoms in an infant are different from those in older children. Usually an infant will be extremely irritable, with prolonged crying, loss of appetite, and high fever (103° to 105°F). Convulsive seizures or extreme drowsiness may occur later.

To prevent complications of meningitis, such as deafness, brain damage, or death, the disease must be diagnosed and treated quickly in a hospital setting. Rapid examination of the spinal fluid by a spinal tap is an absolute necessity.

Symptoms of Viral Meningitis

Symptoms can begin suddenly or gradually after one to five days of incubation. The symptoms include: headache, fever, vomiting, or abdominal pain, followed in a day or two by a stiff neck. Sometimes a rash develops on the body. Children with viral meningitis are also hospitalized, but they completely recover in a few days without antibiotic treatment. The disease is self-limited.

What is a close contact?

When I worked as the director of communicable disease control at the Nassau County Health Department, many cases of meningitis were reported to us each year. Soon after each case was reported, the most frequent question parents asked was about prevention: "My child is a friend (or schoolmate) of that child who has meningitis. Should my child receive antibiotics as a preventive measure?"

The answer to that question was never easy or clear-cut. Like many other local health departments, we used the following guidelines in responding to these parents before we referred them to their own doctor:

Your child may have been in close contact with meningitis if, during the week *before* the meningitis infected person was diagnosed, your child:

- Was a member of the same family or household
- Was in the same day-care or nursery school class
- Sat or stood within three feet of the ill child for at *least* one hour
- Shared food or drink or cigarettes

• Kissed him or wrestled with him

What Parents Can Do

• If your child has a headache, fever, and vomiting and his neck appears stiff, have him examined immediately by your pediatrician or in a nearby hospital emergency room.

• If your infant suddenly develops fever and vomiting along with restlessness and long periods of crying, have him examined by the doctor.

• If your infant or child develops a fever followed by convulsions, bring him to the doctor or nearby emergency room immediately.

• Have your child immunized with the *H. influenzae* vaccine during early infancy.

• If your child has been exposed to another child who has meningitis as a close contact (see above definition), call the doctor. She will advise you whether your child needs antibiotic treatment.

What the Doctor May Do

• In the case of a child who has been exposed to someone with meningitis, the doctor may prescribe an antibiotic as a preventive measure for a short time.

• Delay taking a throat culture in order to clarify the child's exposure status. This is because a throat culture may be positive for someone who is a carrier for meningitis but truly does not have the disease. Therefore, the culture doesn't aid the early diagnosis.

• Hospitalize your child if he has symptoms of meningitis; have a spinal tap done as soon as possible in the hospital (for spinal fluid analysis and culture) and have blood, nose, and throat cultures taken.

• Begin intravenous antibiotics immediately if the spinal fluid shows an abnormal number of white blood cells.

25

MONONUCLEOSIS

Infectious mononucleosis ("mono") looks like many diseases characterized by fever, sore throat, and swollen glands. That's why many adults don't realize they had this illness at a young age. However, "mono" is common, and antibody studies have shown that up to 90 percent of people have had the disease by the time they're adults.

In the underdeveloped countries of the world and among the lower-income populations of the United States, this communicable disease causes a mild illness in many children under three years of age. Often the disease is so mild in these young ones that no symptoms occur at all. These children, nevertheless, develop antibodies to it and become immune for life.

Mononucleosis can affect people at any age. However, when your child reaches high-school age, he will enter the prime time for infectious "mono." With the onset of puberty comes kissing, and with kissing, there is an exchange of saliva. This is the most common way to catch the disease and explains why mono is called "the kissing disease."

Cause

Mononucleosis is caused by the *Epstein-Barr virus* (EBV), one of the herpes virus group. The virus travels in the saliva of an infected person. While the infected saliva is on the hands, food, or toys, it can spread from person to person. Since this virus is not spread through the air like the upper respiratory viruses that cause coughing and sneezing, it is not as contagious.

There's about a 50 percent chance that your child (if he never had mono before) will actually catch it if he's in close contact with a person who has it. This so-called attack rate is much less than the 90 percent rate for chicken pox or measles.

Mononucleosis is around in every season of the year, and it can remain in the throat and saliva and be spread for many months after the illness is over. It also can be carried for months in the saliva of healthy adults who are immune to it (that is, they had the disease years ago but can simply carry the virus in their throat temporarily). They are called healthy carriers of the EBV.

Symptoms

After four to six weeks of incubation, symptoms begin in your child or adolescent either gradually or suddenly. Symptoms can range from none to mild to severe, but usually are mild. Sometimes the illness begins with fatigue, headache, loss of appetite, and abdominal pain for about one or two weeks. Fever may start and rise to 103°F and last for a week or more. In some cases, it can reach 104° to 105° and continue for a couple of weeks. Usually the younger your child, the lower the fever.

The chief complaint of your child with mono will probably be a very sore throat. Then he will develop swollen lymph glands tender to touch, especially in his neck. Lymph glands in his armpits, groin, and elbows may enlarge, too. When the doctor examines his abdomen, she will probably feel an enlarged spleen and liver. Your child's eyelids may become swollen, and a body rash may appear for a short time. It may take days or weeks for the gland swellings to disappear gradually and for him to regain his full strength.

About eight out of 10 children with the disease will have some inflammation of the liver (hepatitis), and sometimes jaundice (yellow skin and eyeballs) develops. The doctor may order blood tests to check on the liver condition.

Mono can look like many other diseases, including strep throat and tonsillitis. Whenever sore throat and fever last for more than one day, bring your child or adolescent to the doctor for a diagnosis. If she finds many swollen lymph glands in the body or if the spleen and liver are enlarged, she will probably advise blood tests for infectious mononucleosis. These tests (antibody and blood count) are the only way to prove the diagnosis of mono in your child.

Very few children or adolescents develop coughing, which might indicate pneumonia, during this illness. Complications that involve the brain or nervous system are also rare.

Although there is no specific treatment for mono, the doctor may advise medications to treat the various symptoms and recommend rest at home for a couple of weeks or so. If your child's spleen is enlarged, he should avoid contact sports (like football or wrestling) until the doctor can no longer feel it on examination. That precaution will prevent the accidental rupture of the spleen.

Your child will probably be free of all symptoms and signs of mono within four weeks. There is a small chance that he may be tired and run fever on and off for a few months. This situation is called chronic mono, but it isn't serious and doesn't cause any permanent harm.

What Parents Can Do

- Bring your child or adolescent to the doctor for an examination whenever he has fever and a sore throat for more than 24 hours.

120

- If your child has mono, he can return to school when he has no fever and the doctor feels he is strong enough to resume normal activities. The doctor may also want to test his liver before making the decision to allow him back.
- If your child's spleen is enlarged, he won't be allowed to play contact sports until the doctor examines his abdomen and determines that this is no longer a problem. Obtain a doctor's note for the school's physical education director. Provide emotional support and reassurance for your child if he needs it. Explain the risk of injuring his spleen during sports and the possibility of requiring emergency surgery.
- Although your child will return to school and all social activities a short time after his mono, he needs to know that the virus (EBV) will remain in his saliva for many months thereafter.
- In order to prevent your child from spreading the virus, urge him to wash his hands frequently each day and not to share food and drinks with his friends. Also remind him that kissing (on the mouth) will be risky for those he may be close to during several months after his illness.

What the Doctor May Do

- Examine your child's throat, abdomen, and lymph glands.
- Order blood tests to determine whether your child has infectious mononucleosis.
- Order blood tests to check on the condition of your child's liver if he is diagnosed with mono.
- Prescribe medication to treat the symptoms, such as sore throat, fever, aches, and pains.

26

~~~~~~

MUMPS

Mumps is a contagious infection and swelling of the salivary glands under or above the jawbone. Years ago, measles, German measles, chickenpox, and mumps were so common that they were known as "the usual childhood diseases." With the great success of the vaccines developed since the 1960s, only chickenpox remains "usual" in the United States, because its vaccine isn't yet available like the others. Children in most developing countries of the world still experience widespread outbreaks of all these diseases because of limited vaccination programs.

Most cases of mumps occur in children from five to 15 years of age, but it can attack susceptible people of any age. The majority of infants are protected against mumps by their mother's antibodies to the disease for several months after birth. As with most communicable diseases, winter and spring are the most likely seasons for developing mumps. Either the mumps vaccine or one attack of the disease itself—even if only a single salivary gland is swollen—will protect a child for her lifetime.

Antibody studies have shown that over 85 percent of adults born before 1957 had mumps as children or adolescents, whether they or their parents knew it or not. They are, therefore, completely immune to it.

In the past, many parents thought their children had mumps two or three times. That misconception was common because swollen lymph glands in the neck can appear whenever a child comes down with almost any type of throat infection. Parents often confused these enlarged glands with the salivary glands that appear along the jawbone in mumps. Unless there's an outbreak of mumps in the community, the diagnosis of mumps can sometimes be difficult.

Cause

Mumps is caused by a virus, known medically as *paramyxovirus*. The virus lives in the nose, mouth, and throat, in addition to the salivary glands, of an infected person. The secretions of these tissues contain the virus particles that enter the air as microscopic droplets when the person sneezes or coughs. The droplets float in the air and can be inhaled later by another person who is nearby. Saliva from an infected child can contaminate an object such as a toy that another child then picks up and puts in his mouth. But overall, mumps is not as contagious as measles or chicken pox.

The virus that is inhaled into the nose or throat soon settles in one or more of the six salivary glands. The virus multiplies, and the infected glands grow larger. The virus also enters the bloodstream, where it can spread to other organs of the body.

The virus can be present in the saliva, nose, and throat of an infected person from six days before the glands begin to enlarge up to nine days afterwards. This is why if your child has mumps, he should not return to school or day care before the tenth day after his glands *first* became swollen.

Symptoms

About 30 percent or more of children with mumps have no symptoms at all. These are called subclinical (without symptoms) cases. After an 18-day incubation period, symptoms such as fever, headache, and loss of appetite begin. But sometimes you may have to wait up to 25 days to see if your child has caught the disease.

Pain, tenderness, and swelling of one of the salivary glands follow 24 hours after the first symptoms appear. Usually one or both of the parotid salivary glands—one on each side of the face—becomes swollen. These glands lie above the jawbone in front of the ears. The other salivary glands below the jawbone may also enlarge.

The pain in the glands worsens when a sick child chews food or drinks citrus juices. The glands are tender when touched, and the temperature may rise to 103° to 104°F for a couple of days when the swelling reaches its maximum. Within a week, the pain and swelling gradually subside. There's also a chance the other salivary glands may then begin to swell.

Complications

Complications develop in a few cases, even if there has been no noticeable swelling of the salivary glands (so-called subclinical cases).

About 10 days or longer after the start of the glandular swelling, a few children develop headache, stiff neck, fever, and drowsiness. This can be mumps meningoencephalitis (inflammation of the brain). Hospitalization is necessary to make the diagnosis by spinal tap and to monitor the course of the illness. Needless to say, this is frightening and upsetting to parents. In very rare cases, deafness can result, but most children who have this illness recover nicely in a few days without any antibiotic treatment.

About 25 percent of male adolescents with mumps develop mumps orchitis (inflammation of one or both testicles) after one week of the disease. Usually only one of the testicles becomes swollen, red, and painful. I remember a male adolescent who had this condition and was extremely worried about sterility. I reassured him that the problem was temporary and that orchitis rarely causes infertility.

A few children come down with mumps pancreatitis (inflammation of the pancreas) about one week into their illness. They have symptoms such as abdominal pain, nausea, and vomiting, but they also recover completely after about a week.

What Parents Can Do

- Have your child receive the live mumps vaccine (which is part of the MMR vaccine) at 15 months of age. He will also need a booster dose of the vaccine before kindergarten or before entering middle school. This vaccine is safe and gives your child at least a 95 percent chance of being protected against mumps for life.
- If your child comes in contact with someone who has mumps and has never had the vaccine or the disease, it's too late to protect him with an injection. Just watch him closely over the next 14 to 25 days after contact for signs of the disease.
- If your child develops mumps, keep him out of day care or school for at least nine days.
- If your child has swelling around his face, ears, or neck, have him examined by the doctor to make the correct diagnosis and advise proper treatment. If your child has the illness, keep a written record of the date and the doctor's name.
- If your child develops a headache, bellyache, vomiting, stiff neck, or drowsiness during his mumps, contact the doctor as soon as possible.

What the Doctor May Do

- Suggest precautions in your child's diet that will prevent pain in the swollen glands. For example, citrus juices such as orange juice can cause pain, as can chewing hard foods.
- Advise medications such as acetaminophen to relieve pain in the glands and reduce fever, if any.
- Advise keeping your child indoors—out of school, day care, or play group—for nine days after the glandular swelling begins.

27

~~~~~~

PINWORMS

Your child, like millions of others around the world, may become infected with pinworms sometime during his childhood. The sight of tiny white worms (about ¼ inch long) wiggling around his anal area can be shocking. But there isn't much to worry about because they usually do little harm except causing itching and irritation in that area.

Regardless of family income and social class, school-aged children experience a high rate of these very communicable parasitic infections. Preschool children have the next highest rate. It's often a family disease, and parents and siblings can easily become infected from the child who has it. Once the parasite is in a member of the household, it's easy to catch. That's why many doctors treat the whole family at the same time even if only one member has symptoms.

Cause

Pinworms are intestinal parasites called *Enterobius*. They spread from human to human but not directly from animal to human. Animal pinworms are of a different species that can't infect humans. People get pinworms from other people.

Here's what happens: The adult female worm deposits eggs around the skin of the child's anus. These eggs are later transferred by his fingers (from scratching the itchy area or wiping it after a bowel movement) to his mouth or to the mouth of another person he contacts. Bedding, clothing, food, toys, or other articles contaminated with these eggs can also spread the infection. The eggs can also mix with ordinary room dust that carries them throughout the house. They can survive and can cause infection for about two weeks. During this time they can be directly inhaled and swallowed or indirectly swallowed from fingers that have touched dust-covered articles.

The swallowed eggs hatch in the small intestine and mature to adulthood in the large intestine in a few weeks. After mating with males, the adult females travel from the rectum out of the anus at night, usually one to two hours after bedtime, and lay their eggs on the skin. If your child later scratches the area, the eggs will get onto his fingernails. If they later get into his mouth, the whole cycle can be repeated again and again until a large population of pinworms develops in his intestines within a few months.

The parasitic infection remains communicable as long as the adult worms remain alive in the intestines.

Symptoms

Many children and adults with pinworms have no symptoms at all but can be carriers of the parasite to others.

The most frequent symptom of pinworm infection is anal itching at night. Itching can be severe enough to interfere with your child's sleep. Daytime itching around the area can cause loss of appetite and irritability. Oozing, red areas of irritation and scratch marks appear around the anus and buttocks. The worms can also travel into the vaginal area and lead to mild inflammation (vaginitis) and itching. At times, you may see worms on the surface of bowel movements.

With a young child, the best way to check for pinworms is to look closely at his anal area about two hours after he falls asleep at night. Keep the room's light off, and use a flashlight to inspect the area after your spread his buttocks apart with your fingers. Look for tiny, white, threadlike worms that move very slightly. Wash your hands afterwards.

An older child recognizes that something is wrong but may be embarrassed and attempt to conceal the problem. If you see him fidgeting or scratching, consider the possibility of pinworms. A supportive, reassuring attitude will help you to gain his cooperation so that you can check for worms.

Whether or not you find any pinworms, call the doctor for his advice. He may want to make the diagnosis by using the adhesive cellophane tape test. In this test, the tape is pressed against the anal area in the early morning and then brought to his office for microscopic search for the pinworm eggs.

If the doctor confirms the diagnosis, he will prescribe a one-dose oral medication. Because recurrences are common, many doctors advise a repeat dose of the medication after two weeks. If there are later recurrences, simultaneous treatment of all family members may be necessary.

Prevention and Control

To reduce the likelihood of a pinworm infection:

- Educate your child and all family members in strict personal hygiene: hand washing before food preparation, before eating, and after using the toilet; cleaning fingernails regularly; no biting of fingernails.
- Change your child's underwear and pajamas daily for at least two weeks after treatment begins. Don't shake them too much, or the eggs may scatter in the room air. Wash them in a washing machine with warm temperature that's at least 130°F.
- After treatment begins, have your child wear underpants under the pajamas every night for two weeks.
- Have your child take daily showers or stand-up baths for two weeks after treatment begins.

- Clean and vacuum-dust all rooms during the two weeks after treatment begins.
- Clean and wash all toys frequently if any child has pinworms.
- All children and adults should wash their hands after playing with the cat or dog in the home if any child has pinworms. (The pinworm eggs can live for a while in the animal's hair after an infected child pets it with his fingers.)
- Keep all toilets—especially seats—clean every day.

What Parents Can Do

- Remember that pinworms are highly catching and can occur in children everywhere in any season.
- Don't panic if you think you found pinworms in your child, and try not to behave as if it is a shameful condition. Reassure your child about it, and call the doctor for the diagnosis and treatment as soon as possible.
- Once a child becomes infected, the pinworm eggs can spread quickly throughout the home, especially by house dust and by articles and food that are handled by your infected child. Pinworms are not caused by a hygiene problem. But once they are in the household, you need to enforce strict personal hygiene among all family members in order to get rid of them.
- After your child is treated, watch closely for any recurrences within a few weeks. If you suspect one, notify the doctor as soon as possible for further treatment.
- Have your child return to his school or day-care center once he is under the doctor's treatment.

What the Doctor May Do

- She may ask you to look for pinworms around your child's anus at night.
- She may give you an adhesive cellophane tape to press against your child's anus in the morning. She will then

129

examine this tape on a microscopic slide to look for pin-worm eggs.

- If you see the worms or the doctor finds the eggs under the microscope, she will treat your child with a special medication. This treatment is usually repeated two weeks later.
- The doctor may want to test everyone in the family for pin-worms.
- She may want to treat everyone in the family with the same medication and repeat it two weeks later.
- She may advise using an ointment or cream for the anal area to relieve the itching.
- She may advise that your child wear underpants beneath his pajamas every night for two weeks.

28

POISON IVY AND CONTACT DERMATITIS

I n the warm months, children love to walk and run in the grass. Some children love to camp out in the woods. Parents need to be aware that these areas sometimes have poisonous vegetation that can cause a very uncomfortable, itchy rash. The harmful weeds and shrubs are poison ivy, poison sumac, and poison oak.

You may be wondering what these plants look like and where they're found. Poison ivy is a three-leafed, green plant that grows like a weed almost everywhere in the United States. Poison sumac has seven to 13 green, paired leaves and grows mostly in the southern United States. Poison oak is a shrub found mainly along the American west coast. One way for you to learn how to identify these plants is to ask your public librarian to find you a book with color pictures of them.

The type of skin rash caused by these harmful weeds and shrubs is called *contact dermatitis*. Contact dermatitis can also be caused by coming in contact with a particular substance one is sensitized to. In that case, it's an allergic reaction. For example, you may use a new laundry detergent and find that when your child wears clothes washed in it, she develops a rash. This can happen even if she does not generally have a problem with allergies.

Cause

Why do some plants and shrubs cause a rash? There's an oily chemical in their leaves, roots, juice, or smoke (if the plant is burned) that irritates the skin of many people. It is a very powerful and durable chemical, and tiny amounts can stick to fingers or get under fingernails and on clothing. Several days later it can still cause a rash when it contacts skin on any part of the body. But the rash itself or the fluid in the blisters do not cause it to spread to other parts of the body. If your child has poison ivy, for example, it will not spread to her friends or to family members. People can get the rash only from their own personal contact with the plant.

The chemical on these plants can also be brought into the house on the hair of your dog or cat, who may have roamed in the woods. If your child then pets them, she can develop the rash on her hands.

After having skin contact with poisonous vegetation, your child becomes sensitized to it. This means that if she has had poison ivy, whenever she contacts it again, the rash will probably recur and be more severe. Some adolescents or adults are partially or completely immune to the chemical in these plants, but they can't rely on this immunity for their whole life. It can change over time.

Symptoms

Skin reactions can begin within a few hours to a few days after contact with the plant. On the area of contact, blisters appear, with intense itching and burning. Often the blisters are along linear streaks, and the area around them is red. Scratching causes the blisters to ooze, and sometimes the skin becomes infected.

You may notice that the itching is aggravated in hot weather and on humid or rainy days. Skin lotions and antiallergic medications (antihistamines and steroids) can be very helpful in relieving the itching. In order to prevent infection, which can result from scratching, cut your child's fingernails short. If the rash is widespread and causing severe discomfort, the doctor may want to examine her.

Your child is more likely to have a mild case if this is the first time she's been exposed to the plant. The symptoms usually subside in a few days. On the other hand, if she's had the rash before, she is more likely to have a severe case, and the symptoms may last up to a few weeks.

Prevention

The first step in prevention is to do some detective work. Look for poison ivy, poison sumac, and poison oak in your own backyard. If you find them there, ask a garden expert about the best methods for getting rid of them. Whatever you do, avoid pulling these plants out with your bare hands, and avoid burning them. It may come as a surprise, but smoke can carry the chemical in these plants and, once the smoke is in the air, it can cause a skin reaction in sensitive people who are nearby.

Keep your toddler away from all underbrush, and remind your older child to walk on cleared paths in the woods whenever possible. It's also wise to dress children in long-sleeved shirts and long pants when they go hiking. Teach your children how to recognize the leaves of these plants so that they can be on the alert and avoid any close contact with them.

If the leaves of the plant accidentally touch your child's hands or exposed legs during a hike, thoroughly wash the areas with soap and water as soon as possible (within an hour is best). It's also a good idea to wash any of her clothing that may have brushed up against the plant.

If your child becomes very sensitive to poison ivy and develops a severe rash every summer, she may benefit from poison ivy desensitization injections each spring. They may not completely prevent the attacks, but they may decrease their severity. Discuss this method with the doctor.

Other Contact Dermatitis

While growing up, your infant or child may become sensitive to many different substances that contact her skin. Most skin rashes are not due to chemical irritations but are allergic skin reactions. However, in some families, children inherit skin cells that react more easily than most to contact with some substances.

The most common causes of rashes are soaps and lotions you apply to the skin of your child. It may take several applications (over a period of days or weeks) for an allergic rash to appear. Some laundry soaps and detergents can also result in contact rashes. Ask the doctor which soaps and detergents are least likely to bring on this type of rash.

What Parents Can Do

- If you're not sure what the leaves of poisonous plants look like, ask your local librarian for a book with color pictures in it so that you can learn how to identify them.
- Don't let your child walk off cleared pathways while you're walking with her near wooded or shrubbed areas. Teach her not to touch any shrubs or plants along the way.
- When your child is old enough to understand, teach her how to recognize poison ivy, poison sumac, and poison oak so that she can stay away from these plants when walking on her own.
- If you think your child has touched or brushed against the leaves of one of these plants, wash the area of skin where there's been contact with soap and water for ten minutes.

Try to do this *within an hour* after she's had contact. Wash her clothing in hot water.

What the Doctor May Do

- Teach you and your child how to recognize these plants and how to avoid them.
- Teach you and your child how to protect exposed parts of her body when she is hiking in wooded areas.
- Ask whether your child has a past history of this type of rash and how severe it was.
- Prescribe cold water compresses or a calamine lotion if it is a mild case.
- Prescribe a steroid cream or an oral steroid medication in a severe case.
- Prescribe an antihistamine to relieve your child's discomfort.

29

~~~~~~

ROSEOLA AND FIFTH DISEASE

Roseola and fifth disease are mild rash diseases. Roseola is a common disease in infants and toddlers, whereas fifth disease occurs more in school-aged children. Even though these diseases are contagious, thre is rarely reason for parents to worry, as children recover nicely within a short time.

Roseola

The following is a typical scenario for roseola: Your baby looks fine and is eating well in the morning and at mid-day. A few hours later, he becomes extremely irritable and develops a fever of 104°F. You rush to the doctor's office but, after a complete examination, she's still unable to make a diagnosis. A few days later, your baby's fever suddenly subsides and a pink spotted rash appears on his body. It's at that point that you learn what's been causing the problem. Your child has roseola.

Roseola is a disease that can frighten you because of the rapid onset of high fever, but rest assured that it is truly a harmless disease. It's so common in infants six to 24 months that almost all children develop a lifelong immunity to it by the time they reach four years of age. Actually, most young children have very mild cases of it. Some have little or no fever, and some never develop a rash. Roseola can occur in infants under three months old or in children over four years old, but this is rare.

Cause of Roseola

A virus in the herpes family called human herpesvirus-6 is responsible for roseola. Although it is a very contagious virus, the exact way that it spreads from one child to another is not known. There is an abundance of this virus floating around in every community of the world.

Symptoms of Roseola

Your baby is most likely to catch roseola in the warm months of the year (spring to fall). After your child comes in contact with the virus, it takes about 10 days for the fever to appear. The fever (102° to 106°F) begins quickly. It's wise to call the doctor when your child has a high fever. She will probably recommend giving your child acetaminophen and washing him in a warm sponge bath to bring down the fever. Although it's unlikely to happen, you should know that a small percentage of infants have convulsive seizures when the fever reaches 104° to 105°F. If your infant has a convulsion, quickly bring him to the nearest hospital emergency room.

After three or four days of continuous high fever, your infant's temperature suddenly return to normal. At the same time, a pink spotted rash appears on his body. It spreads rapidly from his chest and belly to his arms and neck and then fades out completely within a day or so.

I know that when my young granddaughter recently had this illness, my daughter felt tremendous relief once the rash appeared. It was stressful not knowing the cause for the baby's fever and for the change in her disposition, from a happy smiling baby to one that was constantly crying. The rash was a signal that the disease was nothing serious ("just roseola") and that it would soon be over.

The rash is also a signal that the disease is no longer contagious. At this point, you can let your infant have contact with other children.

137

Fifth Disease

In the early part of this century, several of the contagious rash diseases like measles and German measles were given numbers in the medical literature. *Erythema infectiousum* was one of them and became number "five." Since then it has usually been called fifth disease, which is a good thing because the technical name is quite long.

Outbreaks of fifth disease occur in school-aged children in many communities each spring. In some years, there are many more cases than in others. It's usually a very catching but mild disease. More that 50 percent of today's adults had the disease in their childhood and would show the specific antibody to it if their blood were tested.

Even though fifth disease is not usually reason to worry, it can be serious if a pregnant woman who never had it as a child catches it during her pregnancy. Such women have about a 10 percent chance of having either a miscarriage or a very sick newborn infant.

Cause of Fifth Disease

Fifth disease is caused by a virus called the *human parvovirus B19*. It spreads easily from person to person by respiratory secretions (coughing or sneezing). A pregnant mother who has the disease can pass it along to her fetus. It's contagious before the rash appears, but it's not very catching soon after the rash appears.

Symptoms of Fifth Disease

About four to 14 days after your child is exposed to the virus that causes fifth disease, he may develop rosy-red cheeks that look as if they've just been pinched. He may have a slight fever and a runny nose. Within the next four days, red spots appear on his arms and legs and then on other parts of his body. The rash soon becomes blotchy and then takes on a lacelike pattern, especially on his arms. But appearance varies from child to child.

Your child's rash may last for several days up to a week or longer, and it may itch a little. Over the next few weeks (up to six), the rash may fade in and out repeatedly. Sometimes you'll see it , and sometimes you won't. Exposure to sunlight, exercise, emotional upsets, or warm baths can cause it to flare up for many weeks to come. During this time, adolescents with fifth disease may complain of some muscle or joint pain.

Prevention of Fifth Disease

The only preventive measures you can take if your child has fifth disease is to have him cover his mouth when he coughs and sneezes, wash his hands frequently, and avoid sharing eating utensils or food with other members of the household. But these steps are useful only *prior* to his developing the rash, since that is the time he is contagious.

The greatest concern is the danger of passing the illness to a pregnant woman who has not previously had it. Since there is a slight risk that the virus of fifth disease can affect the fetus in the womb, all nonimmune pregnant women should avoid contact with children who have the disease. This precaution applies to schoolteachers, day-care personnel, and hospital personnel who may be pregnant. It also applies to mothers who are pregnant and who have a child with the disease.

As an adult, you have at least a 50-50 chance of being immune to fifth disease. Your obstetrician can arrange for a specific blood test to discover whether you have the protective antibody to it. If you have the antibody, you have permanent immunity to fifth disease. If the test shows that you don't have the antibody, don't panic. Without immunity, the risk of harm to your fetus or newborn when you have a sick child at home is small (probably less than 5 percent). Pregnant schoolteachers or day-care personnel who are susceptible and who are exposed to fifth disease while at work have about a 2 percent risk of harm to their fetus or newborn. It's serious and frightening, but the odds are with you.

What Parents Can Do

- Call the doctor whenever your infant or toddler develops a temperature over 104°F even if you've spoken to her earlier in the day. A high fever is the red flag that indicates your child needs to be examined.
- If your child has roseola, allow him to play with other children again as soon as his rash appears.
- If your child has fifth disease, he can have contact with other children right after his rash appears. He can also have contact with pregnant women at this point since he's no longer contagious. Although his rash may reappear at times over the next few weeks, he won't be contagious when this happens.
- If you're pregnant and your child comes down with fifth disease, ask your obstetrician about testing your blood to find out whether you're immune to the disease.

What the Doctor May Do for Roseola

- Prescribe acetaminophen every four hours to relieve the fever.
- Advise lukewarm sponge baths if your child's temperature is 104°F or higher.
- Advise encouraging more fluid intake throughout the day (juices, gelatin, water).
- Advise dressing your child lightly and having him sleep without a blanket if he has a high fever.

What the Doctor May Do for Fifth Disease

- Prescribe acetaminophen if your child's temperature goes to 101°F or higher.
- Allow your child to attend day care or school after the rash first appears.
- Advise a pregnant woman who was in close contact with a child with fifth disease (a few days before or after the rash first appeared) to take a test to determine her immunity to the illness.

30

~~~~~~

SKIN INFECTIONS

The skin that covers your child's body acts as a mechanical barrier or protective armor against many harmful agents in his environment. Taking good care of his skin is therefore an important preventive measure. Many bacteria normally live on the skin surface and usually do not cause any disease. But if the surface of the skin is cut or scratched, these bacteria and others from the environment can travel to tissues below the skin and cause infections. Most skin infections are not serious and clear up quickly once they are attended to. However, if a skin infection is deep and reaches the bloodstream, it can cause fever and infect other vital organs, such as the bones or the kidneys. This is why it's important to get early treatment for an infection.

The severity of a skin infection and the degree to which it spreads depend on several factors:

- How infectious the specific strain of bacteria is that invaded the skin
- The quantity of bacteria in the invasion
- How strong the child's physical defense system is in fighting off the invading bacteria
- Whether there has been a delay in getting proper treatment for the infection

Most skin infections on the surface heal quickly after you apply antiseptic solutions or antibiotic ointments. You should ask the doctor which ones to keep around the house. Deep or widespread infections usually require antibiotics prescribed by the doctor in her office. If there is any discharge of pus, she may take a culture to see which type of bacteria is involved.

Besides bacteria, fungi (ringworm), parasites (scabies), or a virus (wart) can infect the skin of your child.

In this Key I briefly describe a few of the most common skin infections that occur in childhood.

Impetigo

Impetigo often follows scratches on the skin, such as those that result from an injury or from scratching to relieve the itching of ringworm, scabies, insect bites, or skin allergies. This skin infection most often occurs on the face but can also develop elsewhere. There are two types of bacteria that cause impetigo: *staphylococcus* and *streptococcus*. Your doctor may refer to these names but the way the impetigo looks and the type of treatment your child receives will be pretty much the same regardless of which bacterium causes it.

Impetigo forms yellow crusts and scabs, and sometimes tiny blisters appear. The skin under the crusts and scabs looks red and raw. The watery or yellow discharge (pus) on the skin can spread the infection to other areas nearby, especially if the lesions are rubbed or scratched. Therefore, it's important not to delay bringing your child to the doctor if he has any infection that fits this description.

Impetigo can be caught by others, and it's wise to take preventive measures. Make sure that your child's hands are washed frequently during the day and dried with his own hand towel. Clean and cut his fingernails. After washing or bathing him, wash your own hands thoroughly. Discourage him from touching the food or eating utensils of other family members. Keep your child at home and away from contact with other children until his skin is completely clear. This usually takes at least two days of antibiotic treatment.

Ringworm

The infection known as ringworm gets its name from the ring-shaped lesions that appear on the skin. These lesions have tiny, red blisters or scabs around their borders. The "ring" gradually expands up to one inch or more in diameter and has a clear area in its center. You may notice these lesions on different parts of the body, such as the face, the groin, and the feet. Another sign of ringworm is an itchy, scaly spot on the scalp, sometimes surrounded by a temporary bald patch.

A ringworm infection in the nails causes them to thicken and become chalklike and brittle. Ringworm on the feet can lead to cracking of the skin between the toes, along with tiny, watery blisters. You probably know this very itchy, burning infection as "athlete's foot." Ringworm on the feet occurs more in adolescents than in younger children.

Ringworm is caused by various types of fungi called dermatophytes. It is spread by direct contact with the scalp, skin, or nails of someone who has the infection or by sharing certain articles with that person. For example, scalp ringworm can be spread by using combs, hairbrushes, hats, or hair clips that contain the hairs of an infected person. Shower stalls and floors can be contaminated with a ringworm fungus if someone with *athlete's foot* walks around barefoot in that area.

Ringworm on your family pet should be treated by a veterinarian quickly because it can spread to your children by direct contact. This is an infection that can be spread from animals to people.

Practicing good personal hygiene and avoiding close physical contact with people known to have these infections are the best means of prevention. Teach your child to dry his body (including feet and toes) thoroughly after bathing or showering because ringworm fungi grow in moist areas of the skin. Take your child to the doctor for the correct diagnosis and treatment of these infections as soon as you notice signs of them. Since he will be contagious as long as any lesions remain on his scalp or skin, he should be kept out of gymnasiums and pools until the condition has cleared. Discard any combs, hairbrushes, or hats used by your child just before and during his infection.

Scabies

Scabies is a parasitic disease caused by a tiny insect, a mite named *sarcoptes scabei*. It can occur in all levels of society regardless of income, housing conditions, or personal hygiene practices. Small outbreaks can occur in some schools or day-care centers.

Your child may catch this microscopic mite by having direct contact with the skin of an infected person. The mite works quickly; within a few minutes after contact, it can burrow under the skin. After two to four weeks, a very itchy rash appears as tiny blisters under the skin where there are red burrow tracks. These lesions usually occur around the webs of the fingers, the wrists, the elbows, or the abdomen. The rash is actually an allergic reaction to the mites and the eggs they deposit in the burrows. The idea that these insects are under your child's skin will probably upset you and may even repulse you. But try not to panic, because it's not a difficult problem to get rid of once it's diagnosed and treated properly.

If your child is constantly scratching his body, bring him to the doctor to be checked out. If the doctor suspects scabies, she may take small samples of the skin and either examine them herself under the microscope or send them to a laboratory. Don't worry about taking skin samples from your child because it's not a painful or difficult process. It's done by taking a tiny superficial scraping. Once the diagnosis is confirmed, you will be advised to apply one or two treatments of antiscabies medication to your child's whole body. Since the infection is highly contagious, many doctors recommend that all members of the household be treated with the medication, whether or not they have the rash.

If your child has scabies, you should keep him away from other children until 24 hours after his first treatment. Schools and day-care centers usually request a doctor's note stating the diagnosis and the treatment before your child can return. After a few weeks, watch for a possible recurrence of the scabies, which would require another treatment.

Warts

Almost all warts are caused by a virus called the *human papillomavirus* (HPV). Warts occur in different sizes and shapes and on many different locations on the body. If your child is over two years old, he may develop a common wart on his hands, face, or legs. The wart, which is painless, may be smooth or rough and range from pinhead-sized to pea-sized. Although it won't itch, the child may pick at it anyway and be bothered by its appearance. If the wart is scratched and opens, the fluid that contains the virus particles can spread to other areas and cause new warts. Some children develop a plantar wart on the sole of the foot; this kind of wart is painful.

Warts can spread from person to person by direct skin-to-skin contact. If they're not treated, most of them disappear anyway within a few months or a year. If you want to remove a wart quickly because you don't like the way it looks, take your child to the doctor. He may advise medication to apply to it regularly, or he may recommend another method to remove it. But there is a chance that it will reappear weeks or months later, regardless of which treatment is used.

There's no need to keep your child away from contact with other children if he has a wart. As they grow older, most children develop an antibody against the common wart virus that protects them from these warts in adulthood.

What Parents Can Do

- If your child has itchy skin or scalp lesions (other than mosquito bites) that last more that two days, have him seen by the doctor. Avoid using over-the-counter medications because they change the appearance of the lesions and make the diagnosis more difficult for the doctor.
- Practice and teach good personal hygiene habits in your home, such as frequent handwashing, having separate towels and combs for each family member, not sharing food and eating utensils, and cleaning fingernails regularly.
- If your child has impetigo, keep him away from contact with other children until his skin has completely cleared or until he has had at least two days of antibiotic treatment. If he has ringworm, he should be kept out of the gymnasium or pool. (Send a doctor's note to school.)
- If your child has scabies, he can return to school or day care 24 hours after the initial treatment is given. (Send your doctor's note with him.)
- If your child has warts, reassure him that they are not permanent, but speak with your doctor about having them removed if they are bothersome or painful (such as plantar warts). There is no reason to keep a child with warts away from contact with other children.
- Check your cat or dog regularly for patches of hair loss. If you see any, take him to the veterinarian for diagnosis because the problem may be ringworm, which can easily spread to your child.

What the Doctor May Do

- Teach you how to cleanse your child's skin lesions.
- Prescribe specific antibiotic ointments or lotions to apply to the infected skin lesions.
- Prescribe antibiotics (to be taken by mouth) if the skin infection is widespread and severe.
- Prescribe an antifungal medication for ringworm infection (to be taken by mouth) for a few weeks.
- Prescribe an antihistamine to relieve the itching of ringworm or scabies.
- Treat the wart by daily applications of medication or by freezing or cauterizing it.
- Advise you when it's appropriate to have your child return to normal school or day-care activities.

31

SUNBURN AND
HEAT STROKE

Since ancient times, the sun has been called nature's "great healer." Today, many people worship the sun and consider a suntan to be a sign of health and good looks. But too much of a good thing can cause a problem. Sunburns can be severe in children, and, if they happen often, they can have negative long-term effects.

If your child gets frequent sunburns, especially on the face, she may develop wrinkled and thickened skin later in adulthood. Many cancers of the skin in older adults can be traced to large amounts of direct, outdoor sunlight received as children. This is most apparent in fair-skinned Caucasians who were raised in warm, sunny climates. But children who have dark complexions can also suffer from excessive sunburn and the skin damage it causes.

Causes

When the ultraviolet rays (UVB) of direct outdoor sunlight fall on your child's unprotected skin for a period of time, she'll get a sunburn. Dark skin takes longer to burn than light skin. The strongest rays occur between 10 A.M. and 4 P.M. even if the day is cloudy or hazy, because the invisible UVB rays from the sun can penetrate haze and light clouds to reach the skin.

Some medications, such as sulfa drugs (antibacterial medication) and tetracyclines (antibiotics), make a child's skin burn more easily and more severely. These drugs are called photosensitizing drugs. In some cases, only a few minutes of exposure to the sun can cause extreme sunburn with blisters. If your child is taking any medication, ask the doctor whether it will sensitize her to the sun and, if it does, take extra precautions against sunburn.

Symptoms

Anytime between one and 24 hours after an overdose of sunlight, your child can develop red and warm skin on areas of her body that were exposed and unprotected. Depending on how severe the burn is, she may complain of pain, and her skin may be tender to the touch. It may be uncomfortable for her to lie in her bed. When the sunburn is severe, her skin may also become swollen, and blisters may appear later. If the sunburn is extensive and your child is very uncomfortable, ask the doctor what he recommends to relieve the symptoms.

If large areas of your child's body appear fiery red and hot, she may develop fever, chills, and general weakness. If this is the case, be sure to have the doctor examine her quickly to advise specific treatment similar to that given for any other type of deep burn on the body. It's not common, but it's possible she is having a heat stroke at the same time and needs to be hospitalized.

After about three days, the sunburn symptoms will subside, and after one week or more, the areas of severe sunburn will begin to peel off. For the next couple of weeks these skin areas will be more sensitive to sunlight and will, therefore, need more protection.

Prevention

Sunburn is a condition that is completely preventable and simply requires you to plan ahead and follow through. At the beginning of the summer season (or spring season in warm climates), you should limit your child's time in direct sunlight to less than 30 minutes each day. If she's fair-skinned, this time should be less than 15 minutes each day.

If you have an infant, cover the exposed areas of her skin or keep her in the shade as much as possible. It's very important to remember that sunburn can occur more readily in infants, and even short outdoor exposure to direct summer sunlight can result in severe sunburn.

Gradually increase the amount of time your child is allowed in direct sunlight (about 15 minutes each day for the first two weeks, then by 10 minutes more each day). If she develops a suntan after a couple of weeks, this will act as a partial skin protector. But some children never tan.

Be most cautious when the rays of the sun are at their strongest (10 A.M. to 4 P.M.) and when your child is at the beach or pool. The UVB rays reflect off water and sand and white concrete. That's why they can often reach your child even when she's under an umbrella or large hat.

In the winter, UVB rays can also be strong when they reflect off fresh snow or ice. This can occur even on cloudy and hazy days, especially at the high altitudes of ski resorts. So, if you're a family of skiers, you also need to take precautions.

If your child does not have adequate sunscreen on her skin and plays outdoors for long periods in the midday summer sun, use protective clothing. This means long-sleeved cotton shirts and long cotton pants. A wide-brimmed hat or baseball cap is helpful, too.

The best protection against UVB rays when at the pool or the beach is a sunscreen lotion applied to all exposed parts of your child's body. Until she develops a dark suntan (if she ever does), it's wise to use a sunscreen lotion having a *sun protection factor* (SPF) of at least 15. If she's fair-skinned, use an SPF of 30. Apply the sun lotion evenly about one hour before exposure to the sun, and reapply it every three or four hours if she's frequently in the water. If you have an infant, check with the pharmacist about water-based sunscreen lotions.

If your child is taking medication such as sulfa drugs or tetracycline, keep her completely out of the sun, because sunscreen lotions do not prevent photosensitivity reactions.

Heat Stroke

Heat stroke, also known as *sunstroke*, is a very serious condition that requires immediate medical attention. Fortunately, it occurs infrequently in children. This is how it can happen: If a child plays vigorously outdoors for several hours and the temperature hovers around 95°F, she may come down with heat stroke. She can also get heat stroke if she plays on a hot beach for several hours without cooling off in the water.

Another situation that can lead to heat stroke is leaving an infant or a child for several minutes in a closed car on a hot day. Under these extreme conditions, her body may be unable to lose its own heat fast enough to keep its normal body temperature of 98.6°F.

In heat stroke, your child will become dizzy and weak. Her skin will be very hot, flushed red, and dry, and her breathing will be very rapid. When you take her temperature, it will register between 104° and 106°F. She may also lose consciousness or have a convulsion. Immediately bring her to the nearest emergency room for treatment, because heat stroke can lead to brain damage or death. Hospitalization is required to bring her body temperature down to normal and to monitor her condition closely.

What Parents Can Do

- Remember that serious sunburn or heat stroke can occur in any child regardless of how dark her complexion. With an infant, make sure her exposed skin is always shaded from the sun.

- Unless your child's skin is protected, limit her exposure to the sun to 15 to 30 minutes each day for the first few weeks at the beginning of summer. This sun exposure time can then be increased by about 10 minutes each day. The safest time for outdoor play is before 10 a.m. and after 4 p.m.

- One way to protect your child's skin in early summer is by having her wear long-sleeved cotton shirts and long pants and a brimmed hat or cap when she's outdoors for long periods. If she develops a good tan later in the summer, she'll need less clothing protection.

- Before you take your child to the beach or the pool or skiing in the snow, apply a water-resistant sunscreen lotion (SPF 15-30) on all her exposed skin. If she goes into the water frequently, reapply the lotion every three to four hours.

- If your child develops a severe sunburn or fever, take her to the pediatrician for treatment.

- If your child develops a high fever ($104°$ to $106°F$) along with her sunburn, immediately bring her to the nearest hospital emergency room.

- Keep your child away from any sun exposure if she's taking any tetracycline or sulfa drugs. In these cases, you can't rely on any sunscreen for her protection.

- To prevent heat stroke, never leave your infant or child alone in a closed car on a hot day. Watch her closely at the beach or pool on a hot day. Check her skin temperature every hour. If it feels too hot, cool her off quickly in the water.

What the Doctor May Do for Sunburn

- Advise cool, wet compresses applied continuously to the sunburned areas.
- Suggest acetaminophen for the pain and discomfort.
- Prescribe an antibiotic if any of the burned areas become infected.
- Advise hospitalization if the burn is extremely widespread and severe.

What the Doctor May Do for Heat Stroke

- Advise cool baths and wet compresses continuously until your child's body temperature returns to normal.
- Advise encouraging your child to drink fluids every few minutes.
- Hospitalize your child if her temperature is very high (104°F or above).

32

TONSILLITIS AND
SORE THROATS

During the first year of your child's life, it would be unusual for him to have an acute infection of the throat (called pharyngitis) or tonsils (tonsillitis). These infections occur more often in elementary school children and in preschool children who have an older sibling attending school. However, upper respiratory infections (URIs) from various bacteria and viruses can cause inflammation (redness and swelling) of your child's tonsils and throat at any age. This can also lead to tremendous discomfort for your child.

The tonsils are almond-sized masses on either side of the throat and are part of the body's lymphatic system. They manufacture antibodies and white blood cells, called lymphocytes. Lymphocytes are important because they help fight the many bacteria and viruses that may enter the nose, the mouth, and the throat. Normally the tonsils tend to grow in size from infancy to puberty and then steadily shrink.

Frequent sore throats and tonsillitis are common in young children. Removing the tonsils (tonsillectomy) does not solve the problem. Likewise, large tonsils rarely need surgery unless they interfere with breathing or swallowing. Many studies have shown that children who have tonsillectomies come down with as many sore throat infections as those children who never had the operation. (Also see Key 4 on adenoid and tonsil problems.)

How It Begins

Your child catches sore throats when he comes in close contact with someone carrying a disease-causing bacterium or virus in his nose or throat. The risk of becoming infected is greater indoors when many people are close together, such as at a house party or at school. During cold weather, indoor environments are even riskier because windows are tightly closed and fresh air ventilation is nil or minimal. As a result, the concentration of coughed and sneezed germs (bacteria and viruses) floating in the room air remains high for a long time.

Causes

There are several bacteria and viruses that cause tonsillitis and sore throat. Usually bacterial and viral infections of the tonsils and throat appear the same to the eyes of the examining doctor. That is why he usually takes a throat culture in the office to determine which type of germ is causing the problem. In the meantime, he may start an antibiotic drug while he awaits the laboratory report on the culture. When he sees the report in one or two days, he may continue the same antibiotic, change it, or stop all antibiotics if the infection proves to be viral.

Symptoms

Tonsillitis and sore throats in children produce pain, especially when the child swallows. Infants and very young children do not complain of throat pain. Instead, they may refuse to eat, may vomit, and may develop a fever of 102°F to 105°F.

Preschoolers may complain of abdominal pain without any throat pain. School-aged children may begin with a headache and fever and then develop throat pain after the first day of illness. The pain may range from mild to severe even when the child is not swallowing. Often the neck (near the throat area) is tender to the touch.

Problems

Hemolytic streptococcal bacteria cause one of the most serious types of throat infections, *strep throat*. Strep can occur at any age but is most common in school-aged children. After close contact with a person carrying these bacteria in the nose or throat, there is an incubation period of two to five days before any symptoms begin. Your child may first show a low-grade fever (100°F to 101°F) and a runny nose. In addition to the fever, he may also have loss of appetite and irritability.

Strep throat must be diagnosed by throat culture and treated as soon as possible with penicillin (or another antibiotic if your child is allergic to penicillin) for a minimum of 10 days. Otherwise, it can lead to rheumatic fever, with joint and heart complications, or kidney inflammation. Your child can return to school or day care 24 hours after he begins antibiotic treatment. He won't be contagious then, but make sure he continues to take medication for the *full* 10 days. Otherwise, his strep throat may return.

Scarlet fever is a type of strep throat that is accompanied by a fine red rash (often slightly itchy) that begins in the armpits, the groin, and the neck and then spreads. It occurs one or two days after the sore throat begins and fades in a few days. After a week, peeling and flaking of the skin may occur in many areas. The condition is treated exactly the same way as any other strep throat.

What Parents Can Do

- If you suspect your child has a sore throat, you will have difficulty determining whether it appears red or inflamed. It takes experience to make the diagnosis, and it's better to have the pediatrician examine your child. He may want to take a throat culture.

- Every time your child has a sore throat along with a fever, bring him to the doctor's office within 24 hours to be examined.
- If your child is diagnosed with tonsillitis or sore throat, ask the pediatrician when the child can return to school or day care.
- If the doctor prescribes penicillin (or another antibiotic), keep your child on the medication for the *full* 10 days.

What the Doctor May Do

- Take a throat culture.
- Prescribe an antibiotic right away or wait for the report of the throat culture before prescribing the antibiotic.
- Advise you to increase your child's fluid intake by giving him many cold drinks. Advise feeding your child bland foods such as ice cream, and gelatin and puddings, which are easy to swallow and to digest.

33

URINARY TRACT
INFECTIONS

There may be a time when your child has fever and abdominal pain, but the doctor can't find anything wrong. One of the first tests he orders will probably be a urine analysis to see if there's a urinary tract infection. These infections frequently occur in childhood.

Urinary tract infections (UTIs) can cause fever and pain, and, even though they can easily be treated, they must be taken seriously. Since the urinary tract plays a vital role in getting rid of the body's waste, it's important for your child's health that she be able to void urine adequately and without discomfort.

Urinary tract infections involve the urethra (the tube leading from the bladder to the outside of the body), bladder (cystitis), or the lower kidney are (pyelitis). During the first month of infancy, these infections occur more often in males than in females. However, this pattern is reversed later on. In older infants and children, these infections happen much more frequently in females than in males. *Chronic* urinary tract infections (that is, long-lasting or recurrent UTIs) are more common in older children and in adolescents who are female. *Cystitis* is the most frequent form of UTI, and pyelitis, the least common.

Causes

Some children have congenital abnormalities of the urinary tract, which means that the structure of the bladder, the

159

urethra, or the kidney is abnormal from birth. This can make a child more susceptible to urinary tract infections. The reason for this susceptibility is that some congenital abnormalities in the urinary tract block the normal, free flow of urine from the kidney to the bladder to the urethra. Some of these abnormalities can be inherited. Therefore, if any of your close relatives have had abnormalities of the kidney or bladder since birth, inform the pediatrician. He may wish to include that information in your child's medical record.

Most urinary tract infections are caused by the *E. coli* bacteria that live in the intestines of all humans. It is normal for these bacteria to live there and, ordinarily, they do not cause any problem. UTIs can also be caused by other bacteria, but this happens less often.

Females have a greater tendency to develop UTIs because:

- They have a short urethra
- Their urethral opening is fairly close to their rectum, where many intestinal bacteria exist in the stool.

An important step in preventing UTIs in your daughter is to teach her to wipe properly each time she urinates and each time she moves her bowels. The direction of wiping or cleansing should always be *downward* from the urethra to the anal opening. (Upward strokes of tissue or cloth from the anal area can easily spread bacteria to the urethra and lead to UTIs.)

If you have an infant, practice this technique whenever you change her diapers. And when toilet-training her, teach this important method so it becomes a lifelong habit.

Occasionally, irritants like some bubble bath soaps, laundry soaps, or tight underpants may cause mild urethritis in your daughter. This type of urethritis is more of an irritation than an infection, but, if it persists, it may lead to UTI.

A male infant who isn't circumcised may develop UTIs more often than one who is circumcised. Daily cleaning of your son's penis during infancy helps to prevent these infections.

Some beverages, such as those containing citrus acid (for example, grapefruit, lemon, orange, and lime) or caffeine (for example, cola sodas or tea), may cause frequent urination in your child. But this occurrence is due to irritation or stimulation and is not the result of a urinary tract infection.

Symptoms

What's tricky is that you may not see urinary symptoms in your child even though she may have an infection. This means that you need to be on the alert for other symptoms, especially with infants. When an infant has a UTI, she may not want to eat and may have a fever, diarrhea, or vomiting. She may have abdominal pain, colic, or long crying spells. If your child is over two years old, it's possible that fever and abdominal pains will be her only symptoms. But usually, she will have frequent urination, hurry to urinate, or have pain while she urinates.

When any of the above symptoms lasts for more that one day, bring your child to the doctor for diagnosis and treatment. The doctor may order a blood count to look for an elevated number of white blood cells. In severe UTIs, there is usually an increased number of white blood cells. The doctor will probably order a urinalysis to look for pus cells, blood cells, or protein. If any of these are found in abnormal amounts, he may then order a urine culture to see if any bacteria are present.

These urine tests require a properly collected, fresh urine sample. This is easier to do with an older child, who

161

can understand and cooperate with what's going on. But an infant does not give any forewarning that she's about to urinate. Rest assured that you do not have to use any methods that will cause discomfort. The doctor can provide you with a special urine collection device designed for infants. One method involves using a plastic collection bag with an adhesive. The bag collects the sample of urine after a short time.

You must be careful that the container you use to collect the urine is sparkling clean. I'll never forget how one of my young patients urinated into a jar that his mother had used for storing gelatin. As he urinated, particles of sugar came off the walls of the jar and fell into the urine sample. Certainly, if I hadn't asked the mother about the kind of jar she used, the results of the urinalysis would have been misleading! Your doctor can provide you with a sterile jar.

After collecting the urine at home, you may have to store it in the refrigerator until you are able to bring it to the laboratory or to the doctor's office. A culture and sensitivity report may take two days or longer. In the meantime, the doctor may prescribe an antibiotic if he suspects that your child has a UTI. When the culture and sensitivity report is later received, he may want to change the antibiotic if a more effective one is suggested by the findings.

The doctor will usually prescribe an antibiotic for seven to 14 days. Be sure you complete the entire course of treatment, even if your child's symptoms disappear in a few days. If you don't, the urinary infection may return in a short time. After about one week, the doctor may want to reanalyze your child's urine to see if the infection is clearing. Another urine culture may be done after the course of antibiotic treatment to make certain the urine has become bacteria-free.

Some urinary tract infections recur in a few weeks or months, especially in females. If this happens, the doctor may order special x-ray studies, sonograms, or blood tests to rule out possible abnormalities in the bladder or kidneys. For males, even one UTI may indicate the need for special studies.

Once your child has had a UTI, she should have occasional follow-up urinalyses over the next couple of years. Remember that UTI recurrences can develop without any symptoms. UTIs that aren't treated adequately and that keep recurring over the years may eventually lead to bladder or kidney damage.

What Parents Can Do

- If any close relatives have a history of bladder or kidney abnormalities, inform the doctor during your child's first routine checkup.
- If your child has fever and abdominal pain for more than two hours, take her to the doctor.
- Follow the proper wiping and cleaning technique when changing your daughter's diapers. That is, wipe in a downward direction only. Teach this to your toddler when she becomes toilet-trained.
- If your infant boy is uncircumcised, clean his penis every day. At the first well-baby visit, ask the doctor for instructions.
- If your child develops a urinary infection, *complete the full course of medication* prescribed by the doctor.
- Have your child's urine analyzed periodically during the first couple of years after she's been treated for a UTI.

What the Doctor May Do

- Advise giving your child acetaminophen if her temperature is 101°F or higher.
- Advise encouraging your child to drink more fluids (such as juices, gelatin, or water) throughout the day. Since citrus juices and caffeine (in colas) may cause irritation of the

bladder and urethra, he will probably advise that your child avoid drinking these fluids.

- He will collect a urine sample for analysis and diagnosis. If you have an infant, he will give you a special urine collector.
- He may take a blood sample to see if your child's white blood cell count is elevated.
- He will prescribe an antibiotic for seven to 14 days and then recheck your child's urine to make sure the infection has cleared.
- He will probably advise follow-up urine tests on a regular basis once your child has a urinary tract infection.

34

VISION AND EYE
PROBLEMS

Vision Problems

Having good eyesight is vital to your child's social, mental, and physical development. Children must be able to see properly in order to explore their environment and to learn about their physical capabilities. Impaired vision can interfere with a child's ability to perform tasks involving gross motor coordination (such as playing sports) or fine motor coordination (such as learning to write). A child who is unable to distinguish between shapes and figures will have difficulty reading. A child who sees poorly may lack social confidence and avoid interacting with others.

Few people have perfect eyesight, and most vision problems are correctable when they are taken care of at an early stage. However, even a minor vision problem in childhood can have a serious impact if it's not detected early or treated properly.

Your child's vision steadily develops from infancy to about 10 years of age, even though the most rapid changes occur when he's between one and two years old. At that time, the structure of the eyes and related areas of the brain are developing in leaps and bounds. Many children first show signs of visual difficulty when they enter school. This is because visual acuity (ability to see clearly) is needed for the reading and writing skills taught in school. It is also because mandatory vision screening tests begin in kindergarten.

Your child should have a vision screening test every year from age three until her high school graduation. Many day-care centers and most elementary schools in the United States perform these screenings on all their children each year. If your child fails this simple test, she'll be referred to an eye doctor for a more complete examination of her vision.

In the United States, about one in 500 elementary schoolchildren has a significant degree of defective vision, usually *myopia* (nearsightedness) or *astigmatism* (inability to focus clearly). You may not suspect that your child has a vision problem because she herself may not realize it or complain about it. It is interesting that children often learn to compensate or to adapt to a vision problem. If it's a problem that your child has had for a long time, impaired vision may be the standard that she is accustomed to, and she may not be aware that her vision could be any different than it is.

Sometimes more serious impairments are present from birth that can delay a child's mental and social development. These vision problems are usually caused by *retinopathy* (abnormality of the retina within the rear of the eyeball) or *congenital cataract* (cloudiness of the eye lens). Premature infants with very low birthweight (under three pounds) occasionally have retinopathy caused by a large dose of oxygen received in the nursery incubator. Before the era of the rubella vaccine, many mothers who contracted German measles during the first three months of their pregnancy gave birth to newborns with congenital cataracts. Fortunately, this is now a rare occurrence.

In order to familiarize you with the most common types of vision problems, I will now describe them each in greater detail.

Nearsightedness (Myopia)
Before or during the school years, your child may have difficulty seeing distant objects clearly. In most children, this

difficulty can be detected by early vision screening tests. Nearsightedness, or myopia, is caused by elongation of the eyeball, and heredity is usually responsible for it. The idea that nearsightedness is caused by reading in poor light or by reading too much is an old myth. These reading habits sometimes cause eyestrain or headache, but not myopia.

From childhood through adolescence, myopia usually continues to worsen, and new prescriptions for eyeglasses or contact lenses may be necessary once or twice a year. Therefore, your nearsighted child's vision should be tested at least once a year.

Astigmatism

Astigmatism is another common condition your child may inherit. It causes most objects—near or far—to appear blurred or hazy. Astigmatism may cause your child to fail a vision screening test, but the actual diagnosis of astigmatism requires an examination by an eye doctor. This disturbed vision results from an uneven surface of the cornea (the front surface of the eyeball) and can be corrected with prescription lenses (eyeglasses).

Strabismus (Cross-Eye)

It is easy to confuse strabismus with the occasional wandering of the eyes that normally occurs during the first few weeks of birth. It's also not unusual for an infant (one year or less) to have one eye turn far inward when he looks to his right or left. Most of the time this is due to the flat nasal bridge and wide skin folds along the sides of the nose. When the eyes turn to the far right or the far left, one of the eyes seems to disappear inside the nose skin fold. This is false strabismus (technically called *pseudostrabismus*), and it will disappear as the nasal bridge matures and narrows.

True strabismus results from an imbalance in the eyeball muscles in which one of the muscles in one eye is weak compared with the corresponding muscle in the other eye. There are several variations of this condition, but most often one eye turns inward to the nose regularly.

Strabismus may be a trait that runs in the family, or it may be a congenital abnormality of the eyeball muscles. It appears either at birth or later on. In some cases, it causes double vision, and a child may stumble or overreach objects. As a result, his walking may be delayed. Psychological and social problems can result if this problem is not corrected at an early age. If you see any signs of strabismus, take your child to an eye doctor (ophthalmologist M.D.). Eyeglasses and eye drops may be used in the treatment, and occasionally surgery is recommended before 18 months of age.

After a while, if the condition is untreated, the deviating eye (the cross-eye) may fail to develop good vision. The child may ignore the image he sees in that eye and use only the "good" eye. As a result, he will have a "lazy eye" condition known as *amblyopia*. The vision in the cross-eye can be restored by early treatment, preferably before three years of age. If the eye is left untreated, after five or six years of age, the child may experience a permanent loss of vision in this "lazy eye." Wearing a patch over the good eye and wearing prescription eyeglasses for the "lazy eye" over a long period of time are the usual ways of treating this problem.

In addition to being on the alert for vision problems, it's important to know about some common problems that affect the health of your child's eyes. Two common conditions are blockage of the tear duct and eye infections.

Tear Duct Blockage
The tear duct (nasolacrimal) system develops slowly after birth and continues to develop during the early years of life. This is why newborn babies don't cry with tears.

It's fairly common for young infants to have a blockage in the tear duct, a short canal that normally drains the tears from the surface of the eye into the nasal cavity. Sometimes this duct is delayed in opening. As a result, a few tears roll down the cheek—usually on one side only—for several weeks after birth. Yellow or white discharge or crusts may appear in the inside corner of the involved eye due to a slight infection of the tear duct sac inside the upper nose. This is called *dacrocystitis*. When you see this happening, bring your infant to the doctor for treatment. She may prescribe an antibiotic ointment or eye drops, or she may suggest a method for "milking" the lacrimal (tear duct) sac that you can try at home. This means applying gentle pressure along the tear duct (the upper side of the nose) with a sterile cotton ball. Even though it can be upsetting to have a newborn with any problem, you should keep in mind that this condition usually clears up by six months of age with very little, if any, treatment. Rarely does it require the eye doctor to probe the tear duct with a special instrument, and this procedure is done only after other methods have been tried.

Eye Infections

The most frequent eye infection your child will develop is *conjunctivitis*. This is an infection of the conjuctiva, the membrane covering the eyeball and the lining of the eyelids.

Conjunctivitis is sometimes called "pink eye" because the white of the eye and the inside of the lower lid appear red, with tiny blood vessels running through them. It often begins with a watery, yellow or white discharge along the eyelids and inside the corner of the eye. If your child has this problem, he may complain of burning discomfort and blurred vision. Itching conjunctivitis is usually due to seasonal pollen allergies. (See Key 18 on hay fever and allergic rhinitis.) The best thing to do when you observe these symptoms is to bring your child to the doctor for an examination.

169

Common colds or upper respiratory infections (URIs) often precede conjunctivitis. In some viral infections, such as measles or herpes simplex, this eye condition occurs as one of the initial signs of the illness. Conjunctivitis can also result when a foreign body, such as dust, gets caught inside the eyelid and remains there for a while. A few viruses, such as the *adenovirus*, frequently cause conjunctivitis. Bacteria, especially *H. influenzae* and *pneumonococcus*, also commonly cause conjunctivitis.

Bacterial eye infections are usually very contagious and also spread easily from one eye to the other. Close contact with your child's face and fingers should, therefore, be avoided as much as possible. Be careful with towels, toys, and pillow cases, which can carry his infection to family members or friends. Parents should wash their hands and their child's hands frequently during the first few days of the infection.

A *sty* is a common bacterial infection of the skin glands on the edge of the eyelid. It is painful and is usually caused by *staphylococcus* bacteria. The doctor should examine your child's eyelid for this condition soon after you notice the redness and swelling on the lid margins. She may advise you to apply warm compresses to the eyelid and may prescribe an antibiotic ointment or eye drops.

Keep your child away from contact with other children until he has had a few days of antibiotic treatment of the eye(s) for any bacterial infection. Ask the doctor when he can safely return to school, day care, or play group without running the risk of infecting other children.

What Parents Can Do

• Make sure your child has her first vision screening test at about three years of age. If your child attends day care or nursery school, find out whether the facility conducts vision screening tests. You can also ask the doctor to do it.

- Have your child's vision checked every year (at school or elsewhere) until she graduates from high school.

- If you notice that one of your child's eyes regularly or even occasionally crosses in or out, have the doctor check for strabismus after six months of age.

- If your child's eyes appear bloodshot (red with blood vessels) or have white or yellow discharge in the corners, have the doctor check for possible infection.

- Use good personal hygiene at home (having separate towels for each person, frequently changing towels, washing hands often) if any family member has conjunctivitis.

- If your child is young, keep her away from contact with other children until her eye infection has been effectively treated with the prescribed antibiotic.

- If your young infant has tearing from one eye, yellow or white discharge, or crusts in the corner of the eye(s), have the doctor examine her to determine whether the tear duct is blocked. Discuss treatment options with the doctor.

What the Doctor May Do

- Administer a vision screening test every year beginning at about three years of age.

- Check your child's eye muscle balance regularly after your child reaches six months of age.

- Refer your infant or child to an eye specialist (ophthalmologist) if he fails either of the eye tests listed above.

- Take an eyelid culture if there is a discharge in your child's eyes or if they are very inflamed ("bloodshot").

- Prescribe antibiotic eye drops or ointment if he diagnoses conjunctivitis.

- In the case of an infant with a blocked tear duct, he may demonstrate a way to massage or "milk" the lacrimal sac.

171

35

WHOOPING COUGH

Whooping cough is a highly contagious disease of the respiratory tract. It causes intense coughing for several weeks, with spells of violent coughs followed by a sudden, deep breath. This inhaled breath produces a high-pitched crowing or whooping sound in children. As you can imagine, it's a frightening experience for parents to hear this sound and it's also very upsetting for the child.

Most of the time whooping cough occurs in children under five years old—especially in infants under one year—but children and adults of all ages can come down with it. Whooping cough is potentially a very serious illness and causes death in one out of every 100 children who develop it before one year of age. There is a very effective vaccine for whooping cough, and, if preventive measures are taken, your child will be protected against this disease for a long time.

You may already be familiar with the vaccine for whooping cough, since it is part of the DTP vaccine routinely given to many infants. (Whooping cough, medically known as pertussis, is the "P" in DTP.) Thanks to the widespread use of this vaccine, the number of cases of whooping cough has decreased sharply in the United States since 1950.

In contrast, in areas where the pertussis vaccine has not been widely given to infants and young children the number of reported cases has sharply increased over the past 10 years. The incidence has also risen in countries where the use of the vaccine has declined compared to previous years (for example, in England, Japan, and Sweden).

Cause

Whooping cough is caused by *pertussis* or *parapertussis* bacteria. These bacteria are sprayed into the air in droplets when a person who has the illness coughs. If your child has never been immunized against whooping cough, she has a 90 percent chance of catching it if she's in the same room with a child who is in the early stage of the illness. A child who is sick with whooping cough is most infectious during the first few weeks of illness.

It's also possible that if you or your school-aged children are not completely immunized against this disease, you can pick up the pertussis bacteria from an infected child and carry them back home to your young infant or other children. Put another way, some people can become carriers of the illness without having the disease themselves.

If whooping cough is not treated, it is "catching" for three weeks after the coughing spell begins. But if it is treated with the right antibiotic, it's not possible to spread it after five days. This makes a big difference in terms of the risk an ill child poses to other members of the household, to playmates, and to classmates.

You may be wondering about immunity. One attack of whooping cough gives long-lasting immunity, and second attacks rarely occur. Immunizations with the pertussis vaccine give reliable and long-lasting protection, too, although the immunity tends to decrease as your child grows into adulthood. However, if she does catch the disease when older, it will probably be a mild case.

Symptoms

The start of whooping cough looks like a common cold. The symptoms, which appear seven to 10 days after your child has been infected, include a runny nose, a slight cough, and a low-grade fever (under 101°F). At this early stage, you and the doctor will probably not suspect whooping cough.

However, the cough becomes worse and more frequent over the next couple of weeks. Spells of from five to 20 repetitive coughs occur, followed by the typical whooping sound. This sound is caused by your child as she tries to catch a deep breath through the windpipe in her chest after a long coughing spell.

During each coughing bout, her face may turn red and her lips may turn bluish due to a temporary halt in her normal breathing. Often, at the end of each attack, she'll expel clear mucus and vomit.

Vomiting after a coughing spell is an early clue that she has whooping cough, and you should call the doctor if you notice this happening.

Infants under six months of age usually don't have any whooping sound after their coughing spell, but they may appear to be gagging or choking. This too can be an alarming experience. Do not hesitate to call the doctor quickly.

Children with whooping cough become fatigued by the frequent coughing spells that occur over several weeks. Don't be surprised if your child loses interest in eating and loses weight. She may lose interest in playing and doing the things she ordinarily likes to do. During this stage of the illness, you need to monitor her closely because the whooping cough bacteria or other invading bacteria can cause *pneumonia*.

In a worst-case scenario (which is fortunately uncommon), neurologic damage from lack of oxygen or bleeding in the brain can result from the intense coughing episodes. This can lead to convulsions, paralysis, mental retardation, or fatality. Although these complications rarely occur, there is a greater risk of them in young infants.

The whooping and vomiting gradually subside in two to six weeks. It takes this long even if antibiotic treatment is given. However, antibiotics may reduce symptoms in the first couple of weeks and may prevent spread to others and complications such as pneumonia. After the whooping spells begin, antibiotics may be given only to limit the spread of the disease to others who come in contact with her.

Even after she recovers from pertussis, a chronic cough may continue for several months. Any new upper respiratory infection (URI) during these months of recovery may trigger a coughing spell that sounds like pertussis again. Therefore, it's important for her to avoid other children who have undiagnosed coughing spells while she is recovering.

Cough medicine and increased fluid intake offer some relief from symptoms.

Prevention

This serious disease can be prevented with a vaccine that your infant first receives at two months of age. It must be repeated a few times before she reaches her seventh birthday. It is usually combined with diphtheria (D) and tetanus (T) vaccines in a triple combination known as the *DTP vaccine*. (See the recommended schedule of immunizations in Appendix A.)

Unlike many viral diseases of childhood, immunity to whooping cough is *not* transferred from the mother to the newborn infant. This is why the vaccine is given so early. The vaccine is about 90 percent effective in protecting your child in his early years when the disease can be the most dangerous. It isn't given to children over seven years old because the disease is milder in older children and adolescents.

During the past 15 years, you may have read a lot of publicity about the pertussis vaccine stating that it causes serious brain or neurologic reactions. As a result of these reports, many parents have asked their doctor not to give their children the vaccine. Unfortunately, several large outbreaks of pertussis occurred in those areas (for example, England) where the vaccine had been omitted from routine childhood immunizations. Many complications and deaths were reported among these sick children.

Although you may be worried about what you have heard, large studies in England and the United States since 1976 show that the risks of severe brain or neurologic damage from the pertussis vaccine are extremely small. These reactions may occur in only one in 140,000 doses of the vaccine. Keep in mind that these risks are *much lower* than the risks of brain and neurologic damage that can be caused by the disease itself. The newer, more purified pertussis vaccine that is now available has further reduced the reaction rate.

After carefully reviewing all the available medical data from around the world, the American Academy of Pediatrics has recently concluded that the pertussis vaccine has *not* been proven to cause any brain damage.

Precautions Before Receiving DTP Vaccine

Before your child receives her next dose of DTP vaccine, inform the doctor if any of the following reactions developed within two or three days after her *previous* DTP injection:

- Persistent crying or screaming for three or more hours
- Fever of more than 105°F unexplained by any other cause
- Convulsions

The doctor will then evaluate the facts and decide whether to give the next dose of DTP or to give DT only (omitting the pertussis part). The doctor must also decide whether a child who has a neurologic disorder, such as a history of seizures, should receive the pertussis vaccine or should wait until a later date.

In all these situations, you and the pediatrician must weigh the benefit and the risk of the vaccine against the exposure risk of your child. For example, having an older sibling in school places an infant at an increased risk for catching whooping cough.

What's Done After Exposure to a Case

Your child should be given a DTP "booster" dose as soon as possible if she comes in contact with a child who has whooping cough and she:

- Is under seven years old
- Did not receive her fourth dose of DTP during the previous three years
- Did not have a bad reaction to her previous DTP injection (see precautions listed earlier)

If your child is under seven years old and has not received her fourth dose of DTP within the previous three years, giving her a booster dose after she's been exposed to whooping cough will be less effective in preventing her from catching it than if she had received her inoculations according to the recommended schedule. (See Appendix A.)

Everyone—children and adults alike—who comes in close contact with a child who has whooping cough should be given an antibiotic as a preventive measure. Usually the person who has been exposed takes the antibiotic *erythromycin* for 14 days after his last contact with the sick child. The antibiotic should be taken *regardless* of how many DTP doses the exposed person has had in the past.

What Parents Can Do

- Have your child receive five doses of the triple vaccine (DTP) by the time he enters first grade. The first one should be given at about two months of age.
- Inform the doctor of any fever, crying spells, or seizures that have occurred within two to three days after the previous DTP injection.
- Have the doctor examine your child for any cough that continues for more than five days.
- If your child develops a whooping or choking sound or vomits after a coughing spell, bring her to the doctor as soon as possible. A special nose and throat culture for the pertussis bacteria may have to be taken and sent to the laboratory.
- Call the doctor for advice if you or any of your family members come in close contact with a child who has whooping cough.

What the Doctor May Do

- Take a special throat culture for *pertussis* bacteria.
- Prescribe an antibiotic (erythromycin) for 14 days for your child who has whooping cough.
- Prescribe an antibiotic for 14 days for all members of the household and recommend that anyone who has come in close contact with your sick child call his own doctor for a prescription.
- Alleviate your child's symptoms with cough medicine and acetaminophen. The acetaminophen will help reduce the fever and discomfort.
- Advise hospitalization if your infant or toddler has a severe case of whooping cough with breathing difficulty or exhaustion.

APPENDIX A

IMMUNIZATION SCHEDULE RECOMMENDED BY THE AMERICAN ACADEMY OF PEDIATRICS FOR INFANTS & CHILDREN (1991)

Age	*Immunization*
2 months	DTP (diphtheria-tetanus-pertussis vaccine)
	OPV (oral polio vaccine)
	HbCV (hemophilus b conjugate vaccine)
4 months	DTP
	OPV
	HbCV
6 months	DTP
	HbCV
15 months	MMR (measles-mumps-rubella vaccine)
	HbCV
18 months	DTP
	OPV
4–6 years	DTP
	OPV
11–12 years	MMR
14–16 years	Td (tetanus-diphtheria vaccine)
	(to be repeated every 10 years)

APPENDIX B

RECORD OF MY CHILD'S ILLNESSES

Child's Name: _____

Date of Birth: _____

* Doctor who diagnosed and treated the illness and office location of doctor
** Other than colds and minor illnesses

Date	Age	Name of Doctor*	Illnesses**	Medications	Complications	Reactions to any Medication

APPENDIX C

MEDICAL KIT FOR PARENTS

The following is a list of items that are important to keep at home in case your child becomes ill. I've included some specific brands, but ask your doctor which ones he recommends. It is also a good idea to keep a first-aid chart or book in your medical kit.

Make sure to keep this kit safely out of your child's reach!

Recommended items for an at-home medical kit include:

- Acetaminophen (such as Tylenol®)
- Antiseptic solution (such as hydrogen peroxide or Bactine®)
- Sterile cotton balls
- Ready sterile adhesive strips (such as Band-Aids™)—different sizes
- Sponge (for sponge-bathing infant with high fever)
- Thermometer (rectal for infants and young children, oral for older children)
- Water-soluble lubricant (such as K-Y Jelly®)
- Oral electrolyte solution (a solution of prescribed amounts of sugar and salt, such as Pedialyte®)

- Nose drops and nasal aspirator (a suction bulb that extract mucus) for infants
- Diaper ointment or cream (such as Balmex®)
- Ipecac syrup (to induce vomiting in some poisoning cases)
- Telephone number of the nearest Poison Control Center
- Sunscreen lotion (SPF 15–30)
- Tick repellent (containing less than 30 percent DEET) (see page 105)
- Tweezers and magnifying glass to remove ticks, splinters, etc.

QUESTIONS AND ANSWERS

How does a warm sponge bath bring down my child's fever?

Apply slightly warm-to-the-touch (85°–90°F) water over his entire body continuously with a washcloth or sponge. In about half an hour, his temperature should drop closer to normal as the water evaporates on his skin. *Cold* water, on the other hand, may cause him to shiver, which then tends to raise his body temperature.

Can I use rubbing alcohol to sponge bathe my child if she has a fever?

Never use alcohol sponge baths because alcohol can be absorbed into the skin and may lead to drowsiness or coma.

At what temperature do I call my child's doctor?

That depends on the age of your child, the height of the temperature, and what symptoms he has. All readings of rectal *or* oral thermometers should be taken *after two minutes*. If your infant is under three months of age and has any rectal temperature *over 100°F*, the doctor should examine him as soon as possible—whether he has any symptoms or not. If he's over three months old, you should speak with the doctor if his rectal temperature is *around 101°F*—with or without symptoms. If he's over one year old and has no symptoms despite a temperature *around 101°F*, you can usually wait to see if it lasts 24 hours before you call. But whenever your child (of any age) has a rectal temperature of *102°F or higher*, call the doctor for advice.

If my child suddenly develops a fever but acts perfectly normal, should I contact the doctor right away?

It's a good idea to speak to the doctor for advice. He may suggest that you cool your child with a warm sponge bath and acetaminophen if his temperature is 101°F or more. He may ask you to watch closely over the next 12 to 24 hours to see if any symptoms appear, including coughing, diarrhea, vomiting, sleepiness, poor appetite, rash, earache, bellyache, or long crying spells. If the fever continues *without* any symptoms for 24 hours or more, the doctor may want to examine him anyway.

My child suddenly stops eating and acts drowsy or very irritable for several hours, but he has no fever. Should I call the doctor?

You know your child's normal behavior best. If it changes, there is an underlying reason. Call the doctor, and ask his advice. He may want to examine her, or he may ask you to give him a progress report later.

Why does my child need 10 days of penicillin for a strep infection?

The *streptococcus* bacteria is very hardy, and it takes that long to kill them *completely* when they settle in the nose and throat. After 24 hours of the antibiotic treatment, there are only a few left alive. But if the antibiotic is stopped, these few can soon multiply to large numbers and continue the infection in the nose and throat and elsewhere. It's very important, therefore, to complete the 10 days of the penicillin even if your child has no more fever and has no complaints at all.

Why do some young children come down with more colds and upper respiratory infections (URIs) than others?

The most common reason is that they are exposed to more of the causative bacteria or viruses in their home, nursery school, or day-care center than some other children. For example, if there are older siblings, they can often carry infections back home from their school or friends—especially during cold seasons. In some families, the mother or father may contact colds and URIs at the workplace and bring them home to their young infants and children. Some children have more exposure to URIs in crowded, indoor environments, such as restaurants, parties, and supermarkets during the cold seasons.

How can I tell the difference between a cold and an allergy?

Nasal allergy symptoms usually include a clear discharge from the nose and frequent sneezing that continue for a few weeks or longer. These symptoms occur most often during the spring or summer pollen seasons. They can also occur throughout the year if your child is allergic to molds, dust, or animal dander indoors. Itchy and watery eyes and itchy nose are often present, too. Common colds, on the other hand, usually develop a yellowish and thick nasal discharge after a couple of days, and sneezing subsides by then. Most colds subside within a week.

How can I tell if my child's bellyache is due to a food she ate or to an intestinal infection?

It's often difficult to determine the cause of abdominal pains. Food allergies may be accompanied by diarrhea or hives within a couple of hours after eating the "allergic" food. Intestinal infections (gastroenteritis) often cause vomiting, followed by diarrhea and cramps and occasionally fever.

185

Other members of the family may have the same symptoms about the same time as your child if they have eaten the same bacteria contaminated food or have caught the same intestinal virus. Abdominal pains and diarrhea due to a food allergy disappear in a couple of days after the food is no longer eaten. But pains and diarrhea due to gastroenteritis may continue for many days.

If your child's bellyache lasts for two hours, you should bring her to the doctor for an examination. The doctor will then figure out the correct diagnosis and treatment.

Should I reduce the food intake of my child when he comes down with a cold or upper respiratory infection (URI)?

It's an old grandmother's tale that states: "Feed a cold and starve a fever." If your infant or child has an appetite, let him eat his normal diet if he wishes. Of course, a stuffy nose tends to decrease his sense of smell and his appetite. If he has fever, he may not want to eat much, but food won't hurt him in any way. The important thing is to encourage him to drink juices and other liquids, such as soup and gelatin, in large amounts during the day. These tend to loosen his mucus and lower any fever.

Our house has a hot-air heating system that seems to dry out our noses and throats during the cold months. Does this promote colds and URIs?

Not directly. But if you or your children happen to have just picked up a respiratory virus or bacteria in your nose or throat, you need adequate moisture in your mucous membranes (linings) to help wash away these germs. And if any of you *are* suffering from a cold or URI, breathing moist air will make you more comfortable. Ask the doctor about using a cool-air vaporizer (humidifier) in the bedroom or playroom. Steam humidifiers are not safe because they can cause accidental burns if not used very carefully. You can also install an efficient water humidifier unit in your central hot-air heating system for the cold seasons of the year.

If my child comes down with chickenpox, can I spread it to my friend's children when I visit them?

No. The chickenpox virus can be spread only if your child visits them two days *before* or five days *after* he develops the first pox lesions. In other words, it's spread only by direct, close contact with the sick child.

My nine-month-old child hasn't yet received his measles vaccine. If he should be exposed to a child with measles in the meantime, how can he be protected?

If your doctor can give him the measles vaccine within 72 hours after he was exposed, the vaccine may have time to protect him. Another way is for the doctor to give him a gamma globulin injection anytime during the first six days after his exposure. If he doesn't develop measles within three weeks after either of these injections, he will still need a measles vaccine when he reaches 15 month of age as part of the combined vaccine called MMR (measles-mumps-rubella).

My child tends to develop herpes blisters on his lip whenever I take him to the beach. How can I prevent this?

The most reliable way to prevent his recurrent *herpes labialis* is to apply sunscreen lotion (Sun Protective Factor 25 or greater) on his lips before you get to the beach. Follow the directions on the bottle as to how often it should be repeated—especially if he bathes regularly in the water.

My four-year-old daughter comes down with one infection or another every month or two. Does that mean she has poor resistance or any basic problem?

Average toddlers and preschoolers develop about half a dozen *viral infections* (including colds) each year. Most of these infections are not serious and occur more often in children attending nursery or day care programs. But if your child develops more than one *bacterial infection* (such as a urinary infection or a strep throat) each year, the doctor may want to check her for a possible underlying reason that predisposes her to *bacterial infections*. Be wary of frequent runny-nose-and-coughing "infections" without fever, because these may indicate allergies rather than infections.

My 10-year-old son was treated for a throat infection about a month ago, and I notice that the glands in his upper neck are still large. Is that normal?

Yes. After many bacterial or viral infections, some of the swollen lymph glands (nodes) can remain enlarged for weeks or months. These can often be seen or felt under the jawbone or in the front or the back of the neck. But they shouldn't remain tender when they're touched. If they are sore, have the doctor examine them. Lymph glands are the body's normal defense barriers that become active and large after many types of infection.

SUGGESTED READING
FOR PARENTS

American Academy of Pediatrics. *Caring for Your Baby and Young Child* (Bantam Books, 1991).

Bachman, Judy Lee, *Keys to Dealing with Childhood Allergies* (Barron's Educational Series, 1992).

Eisenberg, A., Murkoff, H., and Hathaway, S. *What to Expect in the First Year* (Workman Publishing, 1989).

Fleisher, Garry *First Aid for Kids* (Barron's Educational Series, 1987).

Sears, William *Your Baby: The First Twelve Months* (Barron's Educational Series, 1989).

Stoppard, Miriam. *Baby and Child, A to Z Handbook* (The Body Press, 1986).

Zuckerman, Pamela *Your Baby: Basic Care and First Aid* (Barron's Educational Series, 1987).

GLOSSARY

Abscess a collection of pus in an infected tissue of the body.

Acetaminophen a non-aspirin type of drug used to reduce fever or relieve pain (Tylenol® is an example).

Acute having a short course (an illness).

Acuity sharpness or clearness, especially of vision.

Adenoid glandular tissue lying between the nose and the throat.

Adolescence the time of life between puberty and maturity.

Allergy a condition of specific sensitivity to one or more substances in the environment; the sensitivity causes a reaction in some part of the body.

Amblyopia decreased visual acuity in one eye without detectable disease of the eye.

Anemia a condition in which the number of red blood cells or the amount of hemoglobin in these cells is less than normal.

Antibiotic an antibacterial or antiviral substance originally derived from molds or bacteria.

Antibody a specific protective substance, such as an immunoglobulin, produced by the body as a reaction to an antigen.

Antigen any substance that when introduced into a tissue of the body, induces antibody formation.

Antihistamine a drug that opposed the action of histamine and is used to treat allergy symptoms.

Aplastic anemia deficiency of blood cells due to depression of the bone marrow.

Appendicitis inflammation of the appendix (small appendage of the large intestine).

Asthma disease of the lung airways, which become narrowed.

Astigmatism a visual problem caused by unequal curvatures on the surfaces of the lens and the cornea.

Attenuated weakened or reduced virulence.

Bacteria single-celled microorganisms that multiply by cell division.

Bacteriocidal causing the death of bacteria.

Bacteriostatic inhibiting or slowing the growth of bacteria.

Booster dose a vaccine dose given at some later time after the initial dose to heighten the body's antibody level.

Botulism a type of food poisoning caused by a toxin produced by *botulinum* bacteria.

Bronchiolitis inflammation of the very tiny airway tubes (bronchioles) in the lungs.

Bronchitis inflammation of the main airway tubes (bronchi) in the lungs.

Bronchodilator a drug that can expand the caliber of the bronchi.

Carrier a person who harbors a specific infectious agent (virus or bacterium) without having symptoms but who can act as a spreader of the infection to other susceptible persons.

Cataract a loss of transparency of the lens of the eye.

Chelation a chemical process used in the removal of lead from the blood.

Chemotherapy the treatment of disease by administering chemical substances or drugs. It usually refers to cancer treatment.

Chronic having long duration (illness).

Congenital existing at or before birth.

Conjunctivitis inflammation of the membrane (conjunctiva) that lines the eyelids and covers the eyeball.

Contact dermatitis sensitivity reaction of the skin due to direct contact with a specific substance.

Contagious communicable from one person to another.

Corticosteroid a chemical (steroid) produced by the adrenal gland and acting as a hormone.

Croup a condition of the larynx (voice box) resulting in hoarseness and noisy breathing.

DEET chemical insect repellent for skin application.

Defecation discharge of a bowel movement (feces or stool).

Dehydration reduction of normal water content in the body's tissues.

Dermatophyte a fungus that causes infections of the skin, hair, or nails.

Disease a disorder of body functions, organs, or systems.

Dormant inactive or resting state; similar to a latent state.

Drug resistance the ability of certain bacteria to withstand specific antibacterial agents.

DTP a combined diphtheria, tetanus, and pertussis vaccine.

EBV Epstein-Barr virus (as cause of infectious mononucleosis).

Electrolyte solution a solution of salt (often mixed with sugar) used to treat dehydration.

Encephalitis inflammation of the brain.

Enuresis, diurnal involuntary loss of urine during the waking hours.

Enuresis, nocturnal involuntary loss of urine during sleep (bed wetting).

Epidemic the occurrence of cases of a disease in a community in excess of the expected frequency.

Erythema infectiosum the disease called "fifth disease."

Erythema migran (EM) the ringlike rash of Lyme disease.

Eustachian tube a small tube connecting the middle ear with the nasopharynx.

Febrile having fever or pertaining to fever.

Fecal impaction An immovable collection of hard stool in the colon or rectum.

Fifth disease contagious rash disease (*erythema infectiosum*).

Flu respiratory disease caused by one of the influenza viruses.

Functional constipation constipation for which no physical abnormality is found as a cause.

Gastroenteritis inflammation of the membrane of the stomach and intestines.

Gamma globulin a type of protein circulating in the blood that has antibody properties and is an essential part of the body's immune system.

H. flu *Hemophilus influenzae* bacteria that cause acute respiratory infections.

Hay fever an allergic disorder of the nose and conjunctivae, also known as allergic rhinitis/conjunctivitis.

HbCV Hemophilus b conjugate vaccine (vaccine against infections caused by the *Hemophilus influenzae* bacteria).

Hemoglobin the red-pigmented protein of the red blood cells that carries oxygen from the lungs to the tissues of the body.

Hemolytic anemia anemia due to the destruction of red blood cells.

Hepatitis inflammation of the liver.

Hereditary transmitted genetically from parent to offspring.

Herpes simplex one class of the viruses of the *Herpesvirus* family.

Herpes an infectious skin disease of blisters on the skin or the mucous membranes that is caused by the herpes simplex virus.

Histamine a strong chemical that can be released in various tissues of the body and cause allergy symptoms.

Immunity resistance to a disease due to the presence of a specific antibody and blood cells that take direct preventive actions against the microorganism that can cause the disease.

Immunization the process of making a person immune to a specific disease.

Immunoglobulin a specific protein that functions as an antibody.

Impetigo a contagious skin infection caused by the staphylococcus or the streptococcus bacteria.

Incontinence (urinary) the inability to retain urine during the day or night.

Incubation period the time interval between the initial contact with an infectious microorganism and the first sign or symptom of the disease.

Infant a child under the age of one year.

Infection invasion of a tissue of the body by a microorganism that can cause a disease.

Inflammation redness, swelling, heat, or pain in a part of the body due to injury or infection.

Intradermal *within* the layers of the skin, as distinct from subcutaneous, which means *beneath* the skin.

Ixodes a class of hard ticks, such as those that can carry the Lyme disease microorganism.

Laryngitis inflammation of the larynx (voice box).

Lesion an injury or abnormality of an organ or tissue.

Low-birth-weight infant an infant who weighs less than 5½ pounds (2500 grams) at birth.

Lymphoid tissue a tissue that contains certain types of white blood cells (lymphocytes).

Lymphocytes a type of white blood cell formed in various tissues of the body and also circulating in the blood.

Meningitis inflammation of the membranes covering the brain and spinal cord.

Microbe a microorganism (germ), especially one that can cause disease.

Microorganism a microscopic organism (microbe), such as one of the viruses or bacteria.

MMR a combined vaccine against measles, mumps, and rubella viruses.

Mucous membrane the inner lining of various structures, such as the lining of the nose, throat, or intestines.

Myopia nearsightedness.

Nasolacrimal duct the small tube connecting the tear duct in the eyelid to the nasal passage.

Nasopharynx the part of the throat behind the nasal passages.

Neonatal relating to the period from birth through the first 28 days of life.

Nit an egg of a head or body louse.

OPV the oral poliomyelitis vaccine.

Orchitis inflammation of the testicle.

Organic of or having to do with a bodily organ.

Otitis externa inflammation of the external ear canal that leads from the eardrum to the open air.

Otitis media inflammation of the middle ear that lies behind the eardrum.

Pancreatitis inflammation of the pancreas, which lies in the upper part of the abdomen.

Pediculosis the state of being infested with lice on the body or in the hair.

Pertussis whooping cough disease.

Pharynx the throat.

Photosensitizer a drug or chemical that makes the skin sensitive to sunlight.

Pica an appetite or craving for substances not fit as food, such as paint or plaster chips.

Plumbism lead poisoning.

Pneumonia inflammation of the lungs.

Preschool age three to five years of age.

Premature infant an infant born before 38 weeks of gestation (pregnancy).

Primary the first in order of time or importance.

Projectile vomiting vomiting in which the stomach contents are propelled with force from the stomach.

Puberty the age at which the reproductive organs become operative and sex characteristics appear.

Pyelitis inflammation or infection in the lower portion of the kidney.

Recessive trait an inherited trait that does not appear in a child unless it is present in the genetic makeup of both the mother and father.

Respiratory relating to breathing or the organs involved in this function, such as the nose, mouth, throat, and lungs.

Retinopathy any disease of the retina.

Reye syndrome a rare, serious illness that affects the brain and liver.

Rhinitis inflammation of the nasal mucous membrane.

Roseola a contagious rash disease of infants and very young children.

Rubella a contagious rash disease known as German measles.

Rubeola a contagious rash disease known as measles.

Scarlet fever a contagious rash disease associated with a streptococcal sore throat.

Scombroid poisoning food poisoning acquired from eating certain types of contaminated fish.

Secondary the second in order of time or importance.

Shingles a painful skin disease caused by the *varicella zoster* virus (the same virus that causes chickenpox).

Sickle-cell anemia an inherited form of anemia in which the red blood cells are crescent-shaped.

Signs abnormalities associated with a disease that are detected by physical examination of the patient.

Sleep apnea cessation of breathing for several seconds during sleep.

196

Sporadic of (disease) occurrence that is not widespread, that is, a disease occurring "here and there."

Spores the reproductive bodies of certain fungi or plants; also, the inactive resistant forms of certain bacteria.

Staph infection infection caused by the *staphylococcus* bacteria.

Sterile free from microorganisms.

Steroid any of a group of chemicals found in various organs of the body, especially including various hormones.

Strabismus crossed eyes.

Strep infection an infection caused by the *streptococcus* bacteria.

Subclinical denoting the early stage of a disease when there are no symptoms present.

Subcutaneous beneath the skin (also called hypodermic).

Susceptible not having immunity or resistance to a particular disease.

Symptoms any abnormal condition, complaint, or behavior of a person that indicates the presence of an illness.

Syndrome a set of signs and symptoms occurring together that form the pattern of a particular disease.

T&A tonsillectomy and adenoidectomy (surgical removal of the tonsils and adenoids).

T cell a type of white blood cell that is a part of the body's immune system.

Toddler a child between one and two years old.

Tonsil an almond-shaped organ on each side of the back of the mouth at the entrance to the throat.

Toxin a poisonous substance.

Urethra a canal leading from the urinary bladder out of the body.

URI upper respiratory infection, such as a common cold (does not include respiratory infections of the lungs and their airway tubes).

UTI urinary tract infection, that is, any infection located anywhere from the kidney to the urethra.

Vaccine any preparation of modified bacteria or virus introduced into the body to produce a protective antibody against a specific disease.

Varicella chicken pox.

Vesicle a small blister on the skin.

Virulence the power of a particular microorganism to damage the tissues of a person it has infected.

Viruses a large group of microorganisms much smaller than bacteria and that can survive only inside living cells.

VZIG varicella-zoster immune globulin, which may be used as a preventive injection against chicken pox under certain circumstances.

Zoster herpes zoster virus, which is the virus that causes shingles and chickenpox.

INDEX